Color Atlas of
CLINICAL DERMATOLOGY

Color Atlas of
CLINICAL DERMATOLOGY

Editor in Chief
Atif Hasnain Kazmi
MBBS (Pb) MCPS (Derm) MD (Pak)
Chairman and Head
Department of Dermatology
King Edward Medical University, Lahore, Pakistan

Co-Editors
Shahbaz Aman
MBBS (Pb) MCPS (Derm) FCPS (Derm)
Associate Professor
Department of Dermatology
King Edward Medical University, Lahore, Pakistan

Muhammad Nadeem
MBBS (Pb) FCPS (Derm)
Assistant Professor
Department of Dermatology
King Edward Medical University, Lahore, Pakistan

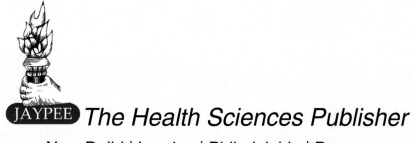

JAYPEE *The Health Sciences Publisher*
New Delhi | London | Philadelphia | Panama

Jaypee Brothers Medical Publishers (P) Ltd

Headquarters

Jaypee Brothers Medical Publishers (P) Ltd
4838/24, Ansari Road, Daryaganj
New Delhi 110 002, India
Phone: +91-11-43574357
Fax: +91-11-43574314
Email: jaypee@jaypeebrothers.com

Overseas Offices

J.P. Medical Ltd
83, Victoria Street, London
SW1H 0HW (UK)
Phone: +44 20 3170 8910
Fax: +44 (0)20 3008 6180
Email: info@jpmedpub.com

Jaypee-Highlights Medical Publishers Inc
City of Knowledge, Bld. 237, Clayton
Panama City, Panama
Phone: +1 507-301-0496
Fax: +1 507-301-0499
Email: cservice@jphmedical.com

Jaypee Medical Inc
The Bourse
111 South Independence Mall East
Suite 835, Philadelphia, PA 19106, USA
Phone: +1 267-519-9789
Email: jpmed.us@gmail.com

Jaypee Brothers Medical Publishers (P) Ltd
17/1-B Babar Road, Block-B, Shaymali
Mohammadpur, Dhaka-1207
Bangladesh
Mobile: +08801912003485
Email: jaypeedhaka@gmail.com

Jaypee Brothers Medical Publishers (P) Ltd
Bhotahity, Kathmandu
Nepal
Phone: +977-9741283608
Email: kathmandu@jaypeebrothers.com

Website: www.jaypeebrothers.com
Website: www.jaypeedigital.com

Inquiries for bulk sales may be solicited at: jaypee@jaypeebrothers.com

Color Atlas of Clinical Dermatology

First Edition: **2015**

ISBN 978-93-5152-627-8

Printed at Replika Press Pvt. Ltd.

Dedicated to

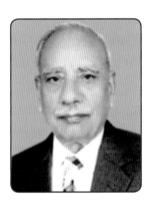

My beloved Father (Late) Prof Ghulam Shabbir,
the Founder of Dermatology in Pakistan, who always
advised and guided me for the progress of the subject

CONTRIBUTORS

Syed Ahmad Ali Gardezi

MBBS (Pb) FCPS (Derm)
Senior Registrar
Department of Dermatology
Mayo Hospital, Lahore
Pakistan

Danish Abbas Kazmi

MBBS (Pb) MRCP (II) UK
Registrar
Department of Dermatology
Mayo Hospital, Lahore
Pakistan

PREFACE

This atlas is intended primarily for medical students, general practitioners, residents in dermatology and internal medicine. Moreover, a color photograph is perhaps the most useful learning material in dermatology. The projection in this atlas of skin diseases on a colored background will aid the physician in making a correct diagnosis. A brief description has been given for an easy interpretation. The book contains 260 colored photographs of various diseases. All the photographs have been taken by our audio-visual section. Most are from patients seen in the outdoor and some are from inpatients admitted in the ward.

This book, in a sense, is a tribute to our teacher Prof Ghulam Shabbir (Late), the Founder of Dermatology in Pakistan. The co-authors, Dr Shahbaz Aman and Dr Muhammad Nadeem's tireless review of the text has made it a remarkable effort. Dr Syed Ahmad Ali Gardezi and Dr Danish Abbas Kazmi generously gave their valuable time and suggestions at every stage; without their inestimable help, this book would not have been completed. We also wish to acknowledge the hard work done by our computer operators Mr Umer and Mr Usman for completing the job efficiently.

The book has also been designed as a study guide to help the medical student or physician learn the subject of dermatology in a way he or she will encounter in daily practice. The color photographs illustrate the differences that lead to a diagnosis. It is our goal that this book serves as the ideal source for medical students, residents or practising physician dermatologists or non-dermatologists.

Atif Hasnain Kazmi
Shahbaz Aman
Muhammad Nadeem

CONTENTS

Chapter 1

INFECTIONS

- **Bacterial**
- **Viral**
- **Fungal**
- **Candidal**
- **Tuberculosis**
- **Sexually Transmitted Diseases**
- **Leprosy**
- **Scabies**
- **Leishmaniasis**

BACTERIAL INFECTIONS

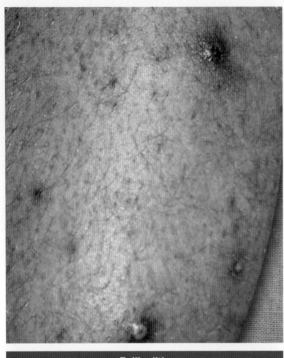

Folliculitis

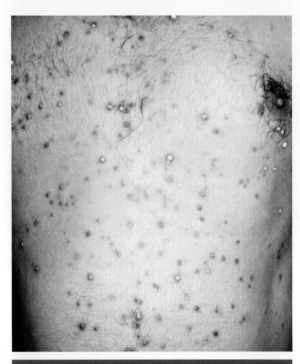

Folliculitis

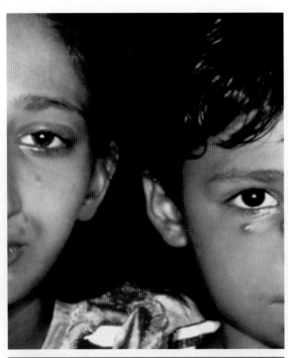

Folliculitis

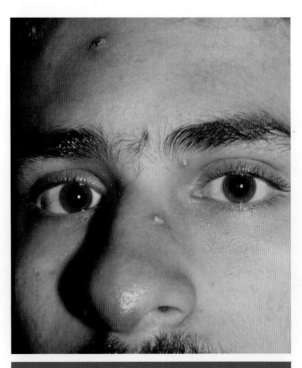

Furunculosis

Bacteria are several types of microscopic or ultramicroscopic single-celled organisms occurring in enormous numbers everywhere in nature. They may be free living, saprophytic or parasitic; some of them are pathogenic to man.

FOLLICULITIS

It is an inflammatory condition of the hair follicle with changes localized to the opening on the surface or extending a little underneath. Causes include bacterial, e.g. staphylococcal; fungal e.g. Trichophyton rubrum; physical, e.g. occlusion with polythene; chemical, e.g. mineral oils, tar; and drugs, e.g. topical steroids. The so called Bockhart's impetigo is a chronic staphylococcal folliculitis. Clinically, it presents generally as painless small-sized papules or pustules around the follicles. Remove underlying cause if possible. Bland local application, e.g. 1% gentian violet or brilliant green paint can be used. Topical and systemic antibiotics can also be used.

FURUNCULOSIS

It presents as an acute necrotic infection of a hair follicle which is commonly seen in adult life particularly in seborrheic individuals and diabetics. Such cases usually carry staphylococci in their noses or perineal regions. Mechanical damage, e.g. friction with collar or belt may determine the site. There is a solitary or multiple, follicular and inflammatory nodules. Soon, the necrotic portion is shed, leaving behind a purplish scar. Tenderness and throbbing is usual. Boils occurring on upper lip or cheek can cause cavernous sinus thrombosis. Treatment includes topical or systemic antibiotics.

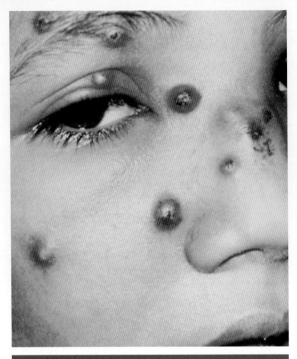

Furunculosis

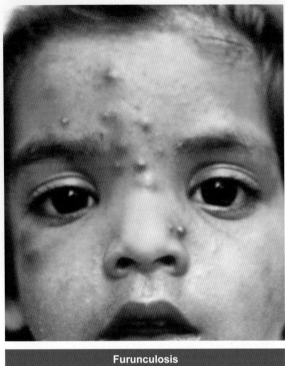

Furunculosis

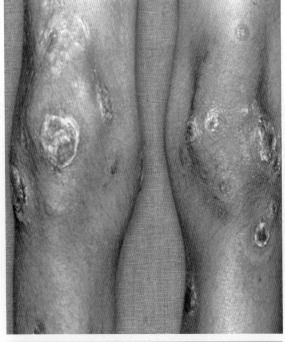
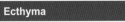

Ecthyma

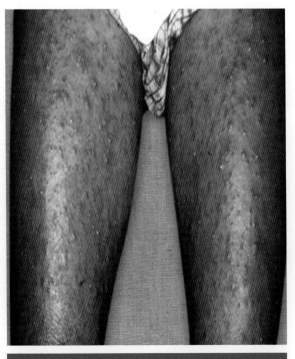

Sycosis

ECTHYMA

It is characterized by ulcers covered by thick crusts. Same bacteria are responsible for it as those of impetigo. Most cases occur in children. Poor hygiene, malnutrition and underlying itchy dermatoses, e.g. scabies and pediculosis are the predisposing factors. Small blisters or pus filled cavities appear on a red base which are readily covered by a thick crust. This crust is removed with great difficulty and the ulcer heals after a few weeks leaving a scar. Commonly affected sites are buttocks, thighs and legs.

SYCOSIS

When the whole depth of a hair follicle is affected by a subacute or chronic pyogenic infection, it is called **Sycosis**. It is seen in males only. Beard region is commonly affected and seborrheic dermatitis is a predisposing factor. Original lesion is a swollen, reddish papule/pustule centered by a hair. The lesions generally remain as such or coalesce to form an edematous plaque studded with pustules. It resembles a ripened fig hence the term sycosis. Recurrent episodes of varying duration often occur without cicatrization. In the scarring variety (called lupoid sycosis), the center is an atrophic scar which is surrounded by active papules and pustules. This variety usually affects the chin, preauricular region or scalp. Rarely, axillary or pubic region, lower legs, thighs or arms may be affected. Differential diagnosis includes ringworm (tinea barbae), lupus vulgaris and discoid lupus erythematosus. Subacute forms are relatively easily controlled by topical antibiotics. A steroid-cum-antibiotic topical preparation may be useful. Systemic minocycline and zinc preparations are also helpful.

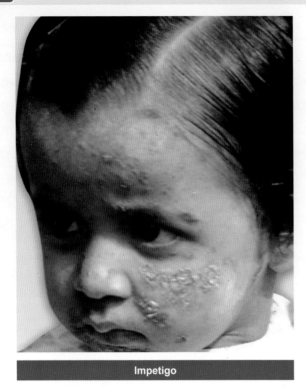

Impetigo

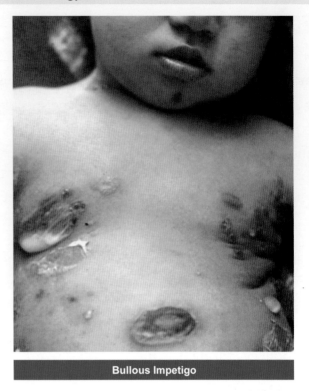

Bullous Impetigo

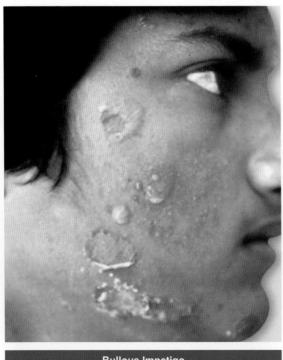

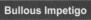

Bullous Impetigo

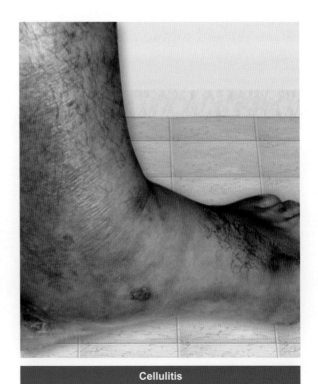

Cellulitis

IMPETIGO (BULLOUS AND NON-BULLOUS)

A contagious superficial infection caused by staphylococcal or streptococcal organisms. Children are most often affected, particularly in summer. It usually complicates an underlying itchy condition, e.g. scabies, pediculosis and miliaria. The so-called pemphigus neonatorum is a form of bullous impetigo seen in infants. There are delicate vesicles principally on exposed parts of the body, e.g. face, hands and knees. These rupture quickly to form golden-yellow or brown crusts. There is gradual, irregular and peripheral extension. Healing occurs without scarring. There are few complications except in the presence of systemic disease or malnutrition. Acute glomerulonephritis may sometimes follow streptococcal impetigo. Differential diagnosis includes seborrheic dermatitis, ringworm, eczema, scabies, pediculosis and pemphigus. Prognosis is mostly good. Topical antibiotic, e.g. neomycin, bacitracin, mupirocin and fusidic acid are used. Usually local applications suffice. Occasionally systemic administration is necessary when cloxacillin or erythromycin should be considered. Crusts must be removed by preparations like starch poultice before applying any local treatment. Underlying dermatosis, e.g. scabies and pediculosis should always be looked for and treated.

CELLULITIS

It is an inflammation of loose connective tissue particularly subcutis, which may be acute, subacute or chronic. It develops most commonly as a complication of an ulcer but can occur in a healthy skin, especially when lymphatic, renal or hypostatic edema is encountered. Apart from streptococci, cellulitis can also be caused by other bacteria, e.g. *Haemophilus influenzae*. Erythema, tenderness and swelling, occasionally bullae can occur. Edge is usually not well defined. Without treatment, focal suppuration, hemorrhagic necrosis and gangrene may occur. Appropriate antibiotic and removal of predisposing factors should be considered, wherever required.

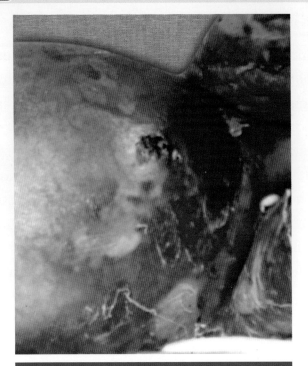

SSSS: Sheets of Desquamation-like a Scald

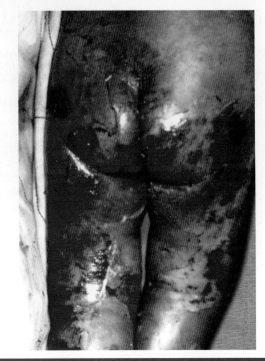

SSSS

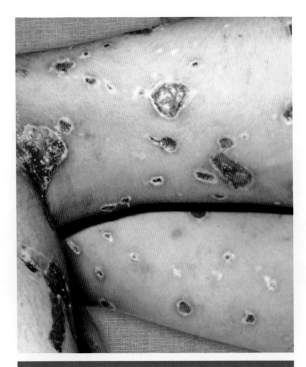

Meningococcemia

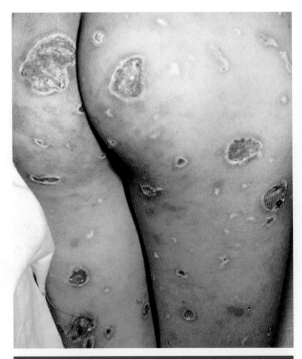

Meningococcemia

STAPHYLOCOCCAL SCALDED SKIN SYNDROME (SSSS)

There is extensive erythema and peeling of the skin in sheets caused by an epidermolytic toxin produced by exotoxin producing strains of *Staph. aureus*. The organisms are not necessarily present on skin but may exist in other sites, e.g. nose, throat, conjunctiva; from where skin is affected presumably through blood. Staphylococci often belong to group-II producing epidermolysin and are usually resistant to penicillin. These organisms may also cause impetigo. Infants and young children are mostly affected but it can occur in adults also. Skin becomes erythematous and extremely tender. Sheets of skin peel off resembling a scald (epidermal separation occurs superficially at the level of stratum granulosum). Trunk, circumoral and genital regions are mainly affected. Unilateral conjunctivitis is common. Differential diagnosis includes burns, SJS and TEN or Lyell's disease. SSSS should be treated with oral flucloxacillin and correction of water and electrolyte loss. Bland local applications, e.g. paraffin gauze and good nursing care are required.

MENINGOCOCCAL INFECTIONS

Acute meningococcal infection is associated with petechial or purpural eruption on the trunk and limbs due to vasculitis or intravascular coagulopathy. The diagnosis is based on direct microscopy of Gram-stained cerebrospinal fluid, blood cultures and culture of cerebrospinal fluid. Treatment is intravenous penicillin or ceftriaxone.

VIRAL INFECTIONS

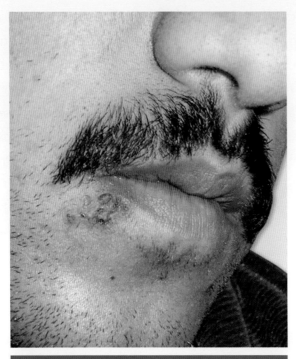

Herpes Simplex

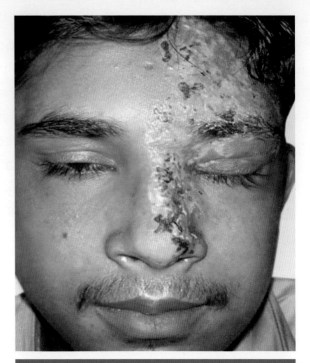

Herpes Zoster

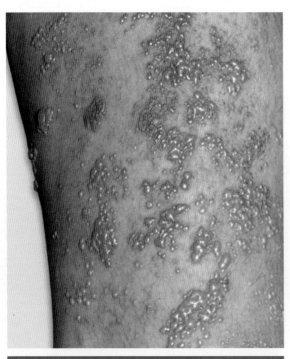

Herpes Zoster

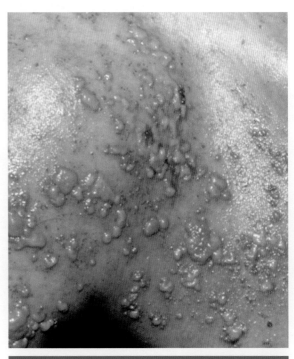

Herpes Zoster

HERPES SIMPLEX

It is an acute cutaneous viral infection, in which one or more groups of vesicles appear on an erythematous and edematous base. The cause is Herpesvirus hominis. Two antigenic types of virus exist: Type I and Type II. It spreads by direct contact or droplet infection. Incubation period is 4–5 days. Over half the cases remain carriers throughout life. Primary infection (herpetic gingivostomatitis) is the commonest. Other manifestations include vulvovaginitis, cervicitis and keratoconjunctivitis. Occasionally viremia causes high fever, encephalitis, hepatitis and widespread herpetic eruption. Recurrent infections are common and are usually precipitated by fever, e.g. malaria and pneumonia, sunlight, menstruation or emotional upsets. In the commonest variety (herpes labialis), clusters of small vesicles occur on circumoral region of face preceded by a tingling sensation. Vesicles dry up and clear usually within a week without scarring. Diagnosis is confirmed by culture of virus from vesicle fluid, examination of paired sera after a period of 1–2 weeks for rise in antibody titre and isolation of virus on electron microscopy or detection of viral antigen by immunofluorescence from the lesions. Spirit and powder are used locally for mild attacks. Acyclovir is used topically or systemically 200 mg five times a day for 5-7 days.

HERPES ZOSTER (SHINGLES)

It is an acute painful viral infection of skin characterized by the formation of grouped blisters on a reddish background along the course of a sensory root. It is the same virus as that of chickenpox. Zoster may give rise to chickenpox in susceptible contacts or vice versa. Conditions lowering resistance, e.g. trauma, malignancy and cytotoxic drugs predispose to herpes zoster. Severe pain in the distribution of a nerve root is often the first symptom. Three to four days later, closely grouped papules appear on an erythematous base, in the distribution of one or more contiguous dermatomes. These quickly transform into vesicles and sometimes pustules. Necrosis occurs in elderly patients and healing usually in 2–3 weeks with scarring. Thoracic region is involved in half of the cases, followed by cervical, trigeminal and lumbosacral dermatomes. In Herpes Ophthalmicus, ophthalmic division of the trigeminal nerve is affected which leads to ocular palsies or even blindness if not treated early.

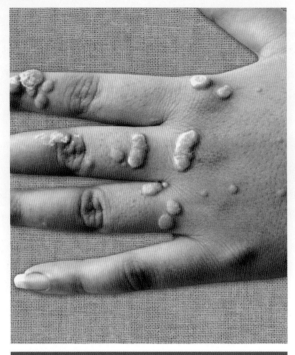

Verrucae Vulgaris

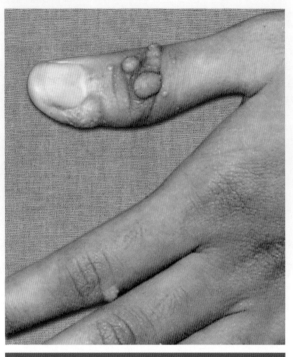

Verrucae Vulgaris

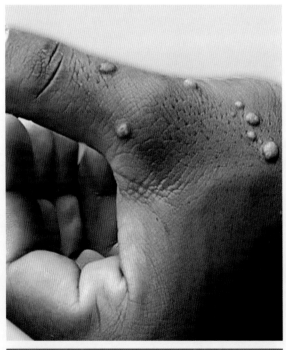

Verrucae Vulgaris

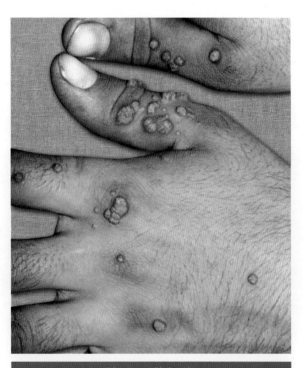

Verrucae Vulgaris

Postherpetic neuralgia is the most serious complication, commonly seen in old age. Pain in the distribution of the affected dermatome is excruciating, intractable and extremely difficult to treat. Problems arise when pain is the sole manifestation. Bed rest, analgesics and local antiseptics are sufficient for mild cases. Acyclovir is prescribed at 800 mg five times a day or valacyclovir 1 g thrice daily for 7–10 days. Hyperimmune gammaglobulin can be used for abnormally susceptible patients. Early ophthalmological opinion should be taken for cases of herpes ophthalmicus. Treatment of postherpetic neuralgia is generally less satisfactory. Drugs, e.g. amitryptyline and doxepin are tried.

WARTS (VERRUCAE)

Warts are common viral tumors acquired by direct contact. Children are particularly prone but can occur at any age. There are following types:

Common Warts (Verrucae Vulgaris)

Usually symptomless cauliflower-like, discrete papules conglomerating into larger masses. Common on back of hands or fingers but can occur anywhere.

Plane Warts

Flat-topped, skin colored or grayish-yellow papules, occurring in clusters on face, knees and back of hands. Occasionally show Koebner's phenomenon. Differential diagnosis includes lichen planus.

Filiform and Digitate Warts

Finger-like projections seen on face, neck or scalp.

Plantar Warts

Usually painful, rounded, hyperkeratotic lesions seen on pressure areas of the soles and occasionally on palms. Plantar warts occur singly on, in clusters. They form mosaic patterns. Differential diagnosis includes corns and callosities.

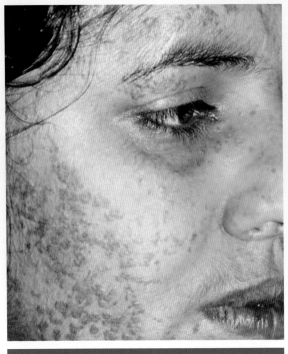

Verruca Plana

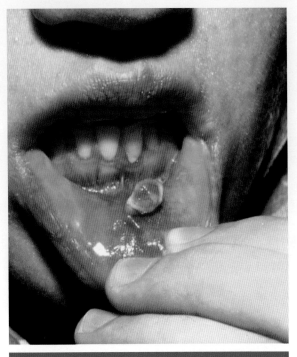

Oral Wart

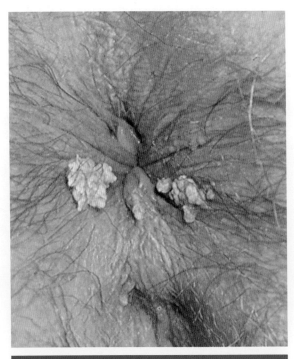

Genital Warts

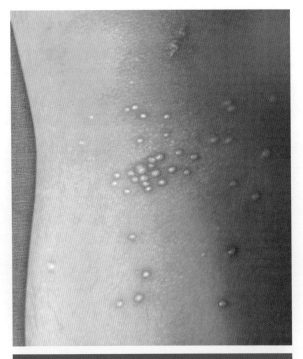

Molluscum Contagiosum

Oral Warts

Oral warts can occur at any place in the mouth or lips. These are usually painless until trauma is encountered. Mostly, small and lying discrete, usually solitary or a small number is found at a single time. They are rough and raised in routine settings, but can appear in a variety of shapes as dome-shaped growths (white or pink like the color of surrounding mucosa), flat-topped papules or thick finger-like projections. Oral warts are becoming more common in our community due to an increase in the oral sex during the past decade.

Acuminate Warts (Condylomata Acuminata)

These are venereally acquired and usually seen around mucocutaneous junctions and intertriginous areas as sessile or pedunculated cauliflower-like excrescences. Maceration occurs commonly, resulting in infection and malodour. Differential diagnosis includes condylomata lata (secondary syphilis).

Treatment

Most warts disappear per se in few months to a couple of years while others are treated with:-
Cryotherapy, e.g. Liquid nitrogen, CO_2 snow; lotion for plantar warts; salicylic acid and lactic acid in flexible collodion, CO_2 laser and electrocautery. Curettage is useful for common, plantar and digitate warts.

MOLLUSCUM CONTAGIOSUM

It is caused by one of the largest viruses known to man and belonging to the pox-group. The disease is acquired by direct contact. Lesions are discrete, pearly white, rounded papules, often multiple with umbilicated centers. Commonly, these are seen on the trunk, face and anogenital region. Individual lesions, on squeezing, yield cheesy material full of viral inclusion bodies. These can be treated with a sharpened wooden probe dipped in phenol or strong tincture iodine.

FUNGAL INFECTIONS

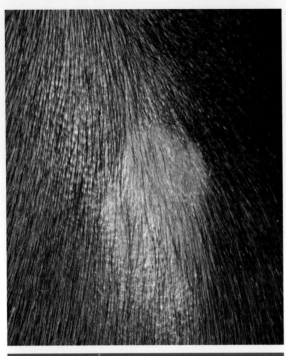

Gray Patch

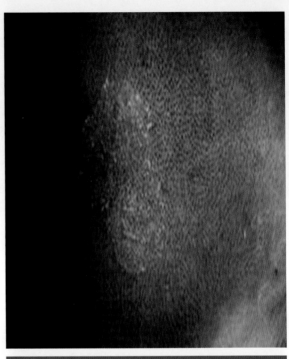

Gray Patch

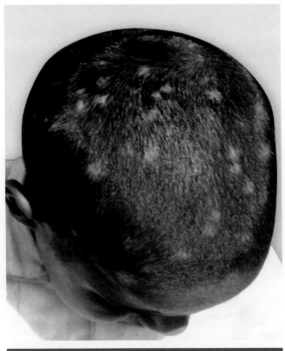

Gray Patch

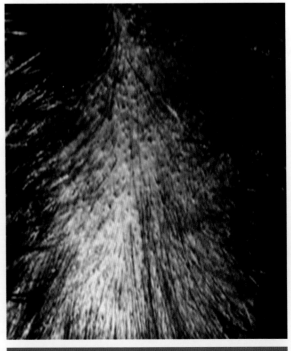

Black Dot

TINEA CAPITIS

Dermatophytic infection of scalp is common in children. Species frequently found include *Trichophyton violaceum*, *T. tonsurans*, *T. mentagrophytes*, *T. schoenleinii*, *Microsporum canis* and *M. gypseum*. Infection is confined to the growing hair. There are five types. The clinical picture depends upon the causative fungus.

Gray Patch: There is an asymmetrical, non-scarring, patchy loss of hair with lusterlessness and scaling. Itching is occasional.

Black Dot Type: In this variety, there is non-scarring patchy alopecia showing black dots representing broken stumps of hair. Usually, it is not itchy.

Kerion: Zoophilic fungi often cause pronounced inflammatory reaction. It is characterized by painful boggy swellings with follicular pustules, resulting in loss of hair and scarring.

Favus: It is caused by *Trichophyton schoenleinii*. Clinically, there are yellow cups surrounding hair, called "scutula" (composed of mycelia and debris). Scalp is erythematous with matting of hair and scarring bald patches. Nails are occasionally affected.

Agminate Folliculitis: In this type, there are pustules with patches of hair loss.

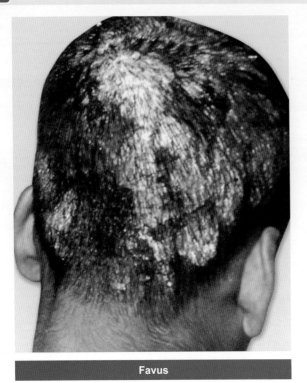

Favus

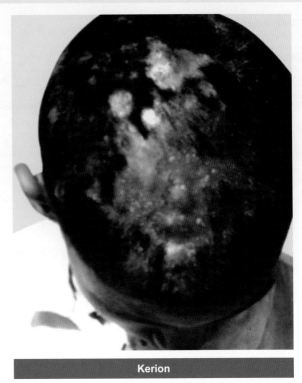

Kerion

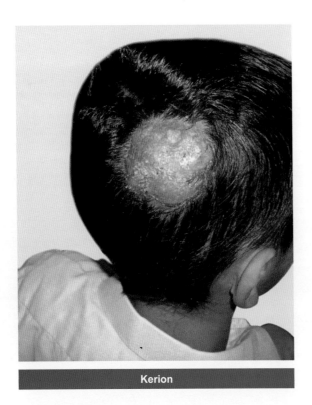

Kerion

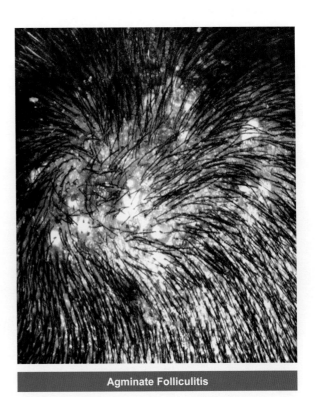

Agminate Folliculitis

Treatment

Topical

Many topical preparations are available, e.g. broad spectrum imidazole compounds such as bifonazole, clotrimazole and isoconazole. In case of secondary bacterial infection, antibiotics can be used.

Systemic

- Griseofulvin tablets: 8–10 mg/kg/day for six weeks to eighteen months depending on the type of fungal infection.
- Terbinafine is fungicidal and well-tolerated. A shorter therapy is required compared to griseofulvin. Daily dose is 250 mg orally for those over 40 Kg body weight and 125 mg for <40 Kg.
- Itraconazole: Broad spectrum triazole compound. It is available in 100 mg capsules. Adult dose is 100 mg twice daily.

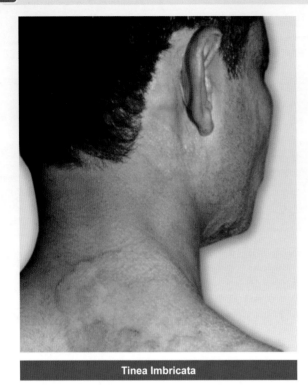

Tinea Imbricata

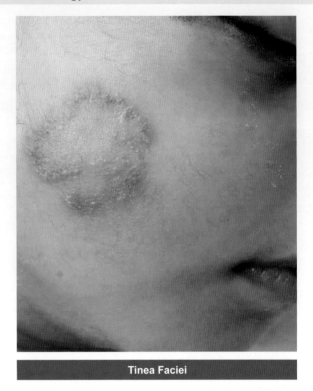

Tinea Faciei

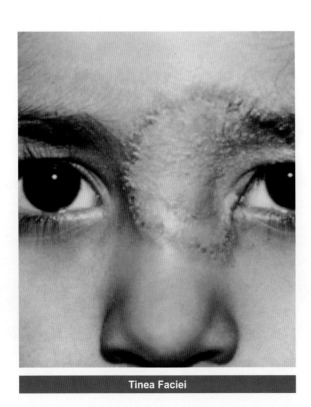

Tinea Faciei

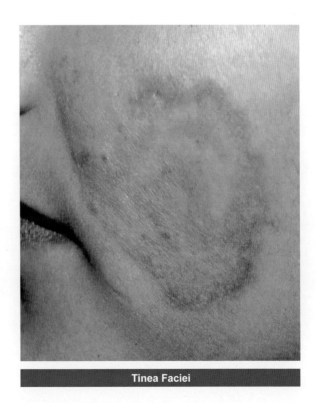

Tinea Faciei

A superficial fungal infection of the skin known as *T. imbricata* or *"Tokelau"*, is limited to Southwest Polynesia, Melanesia, Southeast Asia, India and Central America. Clinically, the lesions are in the form of whirls or multiple rings.

TINEA CORPORIS

T. corporis is a superficial fungal infection affecting the glabrous skin of trunk, limbs and non-hairy parts of the face. Infection may involve terminal hair in these areas. Usually Trichophyton species are involved. It starts as itchy, spherical or oval erythematous plaques with overlying scaling. It spreads in a centrifugal manner. The lesion clears from the center, whereas the active margin is erythematous and slightly raised. It gives rise to a **ring** (annular)-shaped lesion, which gives the disease its characteristic name. Different configurations such as a "flower petal" pattern may be observed when multiple lesions coalesce. Adults taking care of children affected with *T. capitis* (usually the black dot type), may get infected with *T. corporis*. When there is widespread involvement, it should raise the possibility of an underlying immunocompromised state, for example, HIV infection or diabetes mellitus. Differential diagnosis includes psoriasis, seborrheic dermatitis, pityriasis rosea, nummular eczema and impetigo.

T. corporis, often acquired from infected pet animals, is usually extremely pruritic. Athletes especially wrestlers, who have a close intimate contact, can suffer from outbreaks. In such cases, it is called **T. corporis gladiatorum**. Most of them are caused by *T. tonsurans*.

Etiology of Tinea Corporis

The causative organism is a dermatophyte, which normally lives on the superficial skin surface, and when there is an opportunity, it produces the infection. It can also spread through direct contact with an affected person. Humans can also get the infection from animals (especially pet animals like dogs, cats). Sometimes, it is contracted from other animals like cows, horses, pigs, etc. This infection can be acquired by contact with inanimate objects like contaminated combs, hair brushes, bed linen, etc.

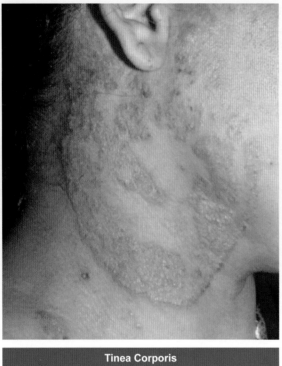

Tinea Corporis

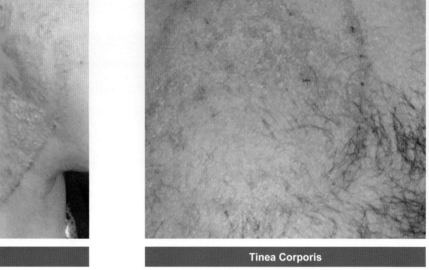

Tinea Corporis

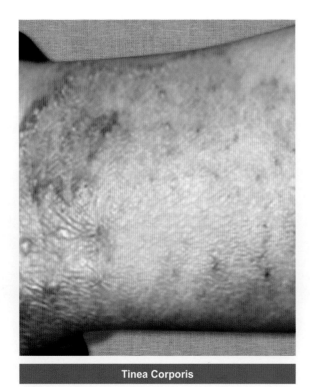

Tinea Corporis

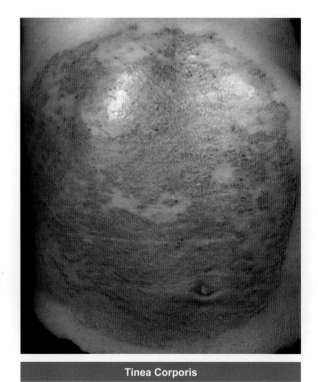

Tinea Corporis

Diagnosis

Once Tinea infection is suspected, the skin should be thoroughly examined and fungal scrapings should be taken. Characteristic segmented hyphae and arthrospores are seen under the microscope, after preparing a KOH mount. For this purpose, material should be obtained from the active margin of the lesion. For confirmation of diagnosis, Sabouraud's medium can be used for cultures. The fungus generally grows slowly, taking several days to show results.

Treatment

Tinea corporis usually responds well to the daily application of topical antifungals. Topical nystatin is ineffective due to its inactivity against dermatophytes. For individuals with extensive cases or patients who are severely immunocompromized, a systemic agent may be preferable. Systemic therapy is also appropriate in patients who have failed to respond to topical therapy. Appropriate systemic agents include oral terbinafine, fluconazole and itraconazole; all of these agents appear to have greater efficacy and fewer side effects than oral griseofulvin. Reasonable regimens in adults include: terbinafine 250 mg daily for one to two weeks; fluconazole 150 mg once weekly for two to four weeks; itraconazole 200 mg daily for one to two weeks; griseofulvin 250 mg three times daily for two weeks.

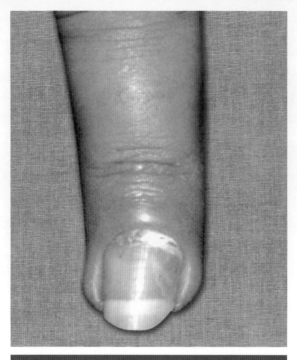

Onychomycosis

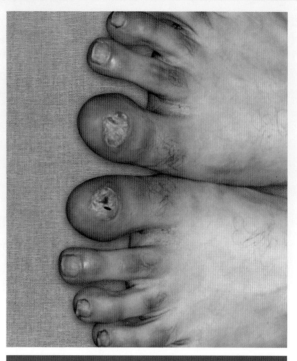

Onychomycosis

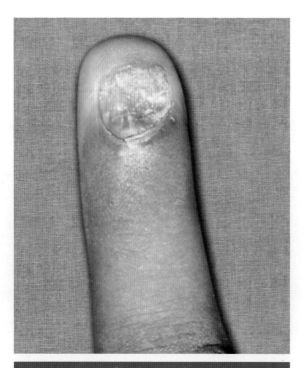

Onychomycosis

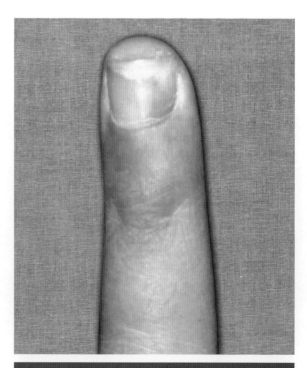

Tinea Unguium

Onychomycosis (ringworm of the nail, Tinea Unguium) is a dermatophytic infection affecting the nail. It is the commonest nail disease and almost half of the nail diseases are due to fungus. It can affect both the finger- and toenails, but infections of the toenails are usually commonly seen. In the adult population, 6-8% prevalence has been noted. A few or all finger- and toenails become discolored, thickened and friable with debris accumulating under their free edges. Four classical types of onychomycosis have been described: ***Distal subungual onychomycosis* (DSO)** is the commonest variety, mostly due to Trichophyton rubrum, which affects the nail bed and the hyponychium. ***White superficial onychomycosis* (WSO)** is characterized by the formation of white islands on the plate due to fungal infection of its superficial layers. It is not a common disease, it accounting for only 10% cases of onychomycosis. Sometimes, ***"keratin granulations"***, produced by the nail polish can give rise to a chalky white discoloration. The diagnosis should be confirmed by laboratory tests.

When the fungus enters through the proximal nail fold, invading the freshly formed nail plate, it is known as ***Proximal subungual onychomycosis* (PSO)**. This variety is rarely seen, but is a common form of presentation in the immunocompromised cases. ***Candidal infection of the nail*** generally occurs in those engaged in wet work. Usually, the organism attacks an already damaged nail (either by trauma or infection). Diagnostic confusions can arise in cases of nail involvement in lichen planus, psoriasis, chronic paronychia, etc. In limited diseases, topical antifungals are only required while in cases of severe involvement, oral antifungals have to be used.

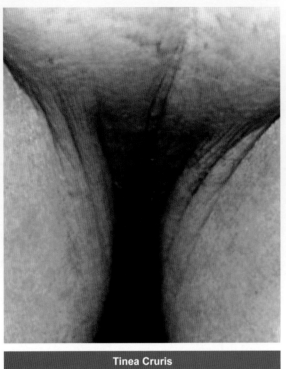

Tinea Cruris

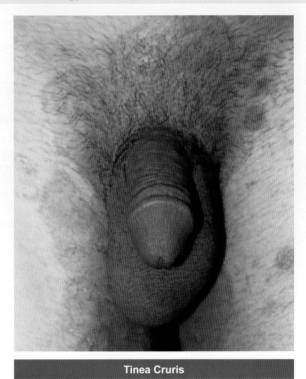

Tinea Cruris

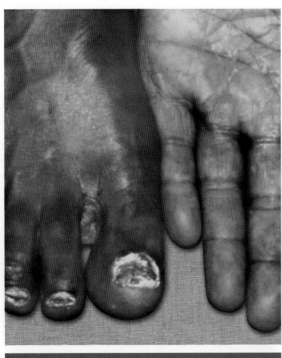

Tinea Manum and Tinea Unguium

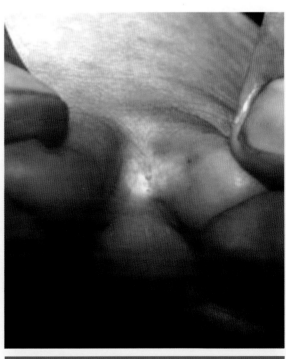

Tinea Pedis

TINEA CRURIS

Tinea cruris is dermatophytic infection of the groins. *Trichophyton rubrum* and *Epidermophyton floccosum* are the main causative organisms. Males are commonly affected, mainly adults. Transmission is by infected clothes and towels. Symmetrically spreading erythematous and scaly patches with papular or vesicular edges are seen. Sites of involvement are thighs, perineum, perianal region and scrotum. The patient often gets infection from his/ her own tinea pedis or tinea unguium, usually following an exercise leading to profuse sweating. Obesity, diabetes and immunodeficiency predispose to this fungal infection. Diseases to be included in the differentials include erythrasma, seborrheic dermatitis, candidal intertrigo and psoriasis. Lab investigation can confirm the diagnosis. A candidal infection is characterized by the satellite lesions. A KOH preparation would easily yield hyphae, pseudohyphae, or yeast. A coral red fluorescence on Wood's lamp examination confirms the presence of erythrasma. In cases of seborrheic dermatitis or psoriasis, similar lesions at other sites help in the final diagnosis.

TINEA MANUM

Fungal infection of the hand is called **Tinea manum**. The symptoms are generally severe as compared to T. pedis. There is marked itching and burning along with dryness and fissuring at times.

TINEA PEDIS

Tinea pedis also known as **Athlete's foot**, is the fungal infection of feet, often associated with dermatophyte infection of the hands, nails or groin.

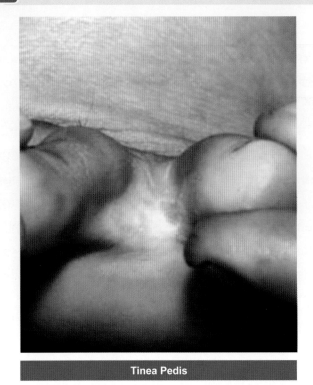

Tinea Pedis

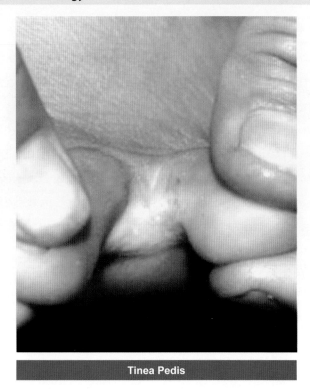

Tinea Pedis

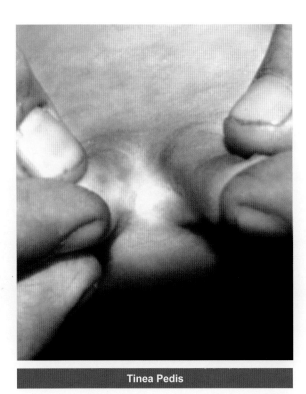

Tinea Pedis

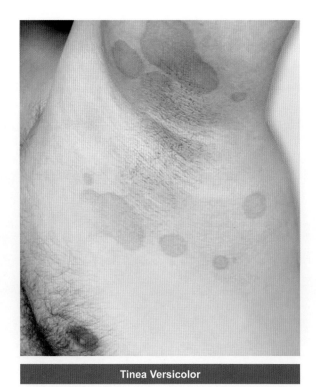

Tinea Versicolor

T. pedis can present in an acute or chronic form. The infection is contagious and is acquired from contaminated floors of communal places. The causative organism in acute cases is Trichophyton mentagrophytes var. interdigitale, while in chronic cases, the culprit agent is Trichophyton rubrum. It may affect one or both feet at the same time. Secondary bacterial infection is common with lymphangitis as the usual complication. Sometimes, the body produces a severe immunologic reaction to the organism. In such cases, eruptions at sites away from the primary area, may appear. This eruption does not contain the fungus and generally develops on the palms and fingers, known as a *id* or *ide* eruption. It clears when the primary fungal infection is successfully treated.

Treatment

Treatment of T. pedis includes topical as well as oral antifungals. Interdigital infection mostly clears with one week application of a topical antifungal cream. Those suffering from extensive infection, may need oral therapy which may be given in the form of terbinafine 250 mg/ day for 02 weeks, itraconazole 400 mg/ day for 01 week, fluconazole 150 mg weekly for 4–6 weeks. If there is nail involvement, it is a further indication for oral antifungal therapy. Oral antibiotics are required for secondary bacterial infections. Other supportive treatments include the use of talcum powder to combat maceration, treating the footwear with antifungal powders, and avoidance of wearing closed shoes.

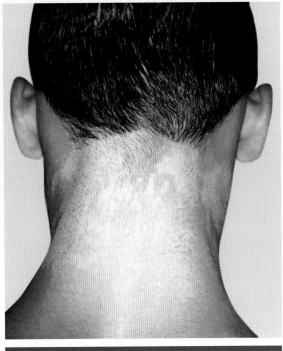

Tinea Versicolor

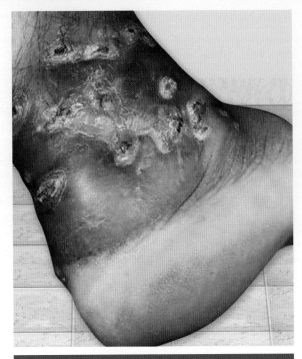

Actinomycetoma: Multiple Nodules and Sinuses with Swelling

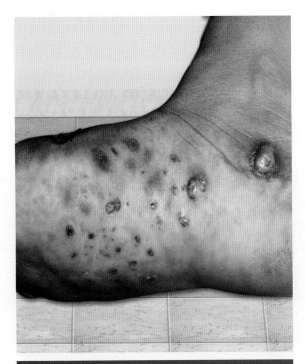

Eumycetoma: Swelling with Multiple Sinuses and Nodules

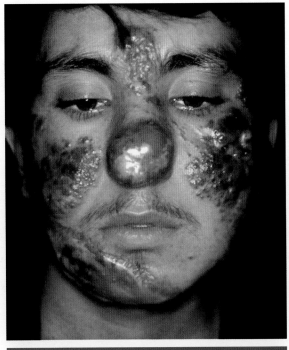

Chromoblastomycosis

TINEA VERSICOLOR

Tinea versicolor (Pityriasis Versicolor) is a type of fungal infection, usually caused by a yeast that is a natural inhabitant of the skin. Any one of these conditions can precipitate this infection: sweating, hot climate, oily skin and immunodeficiency. Because the causative organism lives naturally on the skin, this infection is not contagious. People of any type of skin color can be infected with this yeast, mostly in their teens or young adult life. The disease may manifest as: white, pink, red, or brown patches that may be lighter or darker than the surrounding skin. These patches usually occur on the upper half of body including the neck, front and back of chest, and arms. A fluorescent yellow-green color will appear when examined under Wood's lamp. Treatment consists of topical antifungals, which are available as cream, lotion, foam, soap or shampoo. Oral antifungal drugs can also be given to treat severe infection.

MYCETOMA

Mycetoma is a chronic, localized deep infection. The causative organisms are various species of actinomycetes or fungi. The skin of feet along with its subcutaneous tissues, sometimes even upto the bones, is damaged and there is a discharge of grains from the draining sinuses. **Actinomycetoma** is the bacterial form, while **Eumycetoma** is caused by fungi. Grains consist of collections of the micro-organisms. It was initially named Madura foot, because it was identified in Madura which is a town in India. Most commonly affected areas are the foot or lower leg, mostly the forefoot at its dorsal aspect. This infection usually occurs in villagers, often farmers or shepherds. The **treatment** consists of an antibiotic or antifungal which should be tried initially because it may have to be followed by surgery, especially when eumycetoma is present on the extremities. Localized lesions can be best excised, while a surgical de-bulking of the larger lesions can help improve the response to oral therapy.

CHROMOBLASTOMYCOSIS

Chromoblastomycosis is a chronic, long lasting subcutaneous fungal infection. People in the rural areas of tropical or subtropical climates are the usual victims. Many types of fungal organisms are implicated as the cause, which get an entry into the skin through splinters or thorns. The disease has a slowly progressive nature but is rarely fatal with a good prognosis. It is very difficult to cure Chromoblastomycosis. Various therapeutic options are itraconazole either alone or with flucytosine, terbinafine, amphotericin B and cryosurgery with liquid nitrogen.

CANDIDAL INFECTIONS

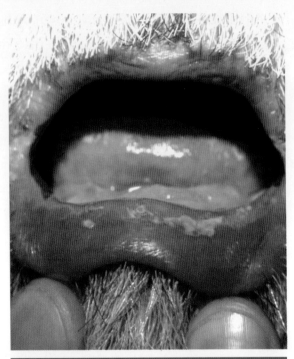

Candidiasis

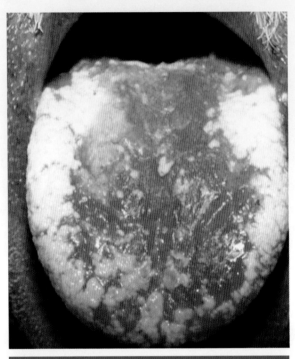

Candidiasis (Oral Thrush)

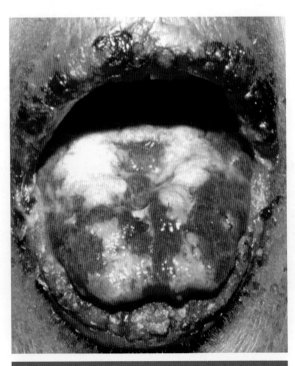

Oral Ulcers with Candidiasis (Oral Thrush): White Plaques

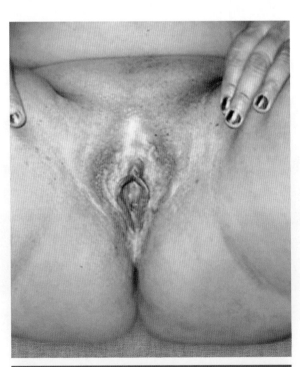

Vaginal Cadidiasis: White Plaques with Erythema

CANDIDIASIS

Candidiasis (Candidosis) is infection of the skin and mucous membranes by yeasts of the genus Candida. Most often the mucous membrane involvement shows up as a thick, white, curdy material covering the glossal, labial or buccal mucosa. There is consequently altered taste sensation and a feeling of soreness. In cases of vaginal candidosis, a similar whitish material may take the form of a discharge from the introitus and involve the adjoining skin. There is itching, burning, and dyspareunia. Prolonged candidal infection can lead to atrophic vaginitis. Cutaneous candidiasis generally involves the folds especially their deepest parts. It presents as brick-red papules and plaques which may be studded with whitish pustules. Small satellite lesions may be seen near the primary infections. It is generally associated with warm, moist environments. An underlying immunocompromized state due to any cause predisposes to candidiasis, such as diabetes mellitus, Cushing's disease, various polyendocrinopathies, anticancer chemotherapy, HIV/AIDS, etc. Even topical application of steroids for oral aphthosis or oral lichen planus can result in candidiasis. Occasionally deeper infections resulting in septicemia, endocarditis or meningitis may occur.

The various **clinical patterns** of involvement include two types of acute presentations like pseudomembranous or erythematous, and various chronic forms, such as pseudomembranous, erythematous, atrophic, plaque-like, nodular, angular cheilitis, and median rhomboid glossitis. Integumentary varieties of candidiasis are candida intertrigo, vulvovaginitis, perianal and scrotal candidiasis, napkin candidiasis, and candidal paronychia. Diagnosis of candida requires microscopy of smears from the affected area which yields yeasts and filaments, due to pseudohyphae or true hyphae.

Treatment

Treatment involves removal of the microenvironment conducive to candidal overgrowth. This may require control of diabetes, reduction in serum cortisol levels if high, removal of dentures or other prosthetic devices, or institution of HAART therapy in patients with HIV/ AIDS. Candidal infections respond to topical nystatin or miconazole, clotrimazole, isoconazole, voriconazole, etc. If recalcitrant and in immunocompromized patients, oral fluconazole or itraconazole may be needed. In chronic mucocutaneous candidiasis, intravenous amphotericin B or flucytosine can be used.

TUBERCULOSIS

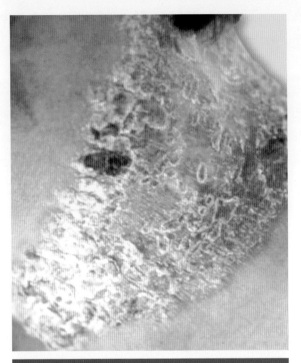

Lupus Vulgaris

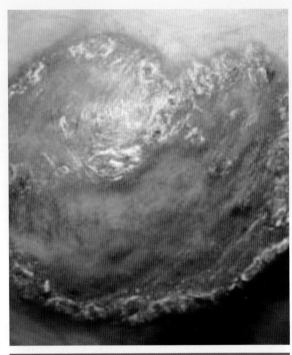

Lupus Vulgaris

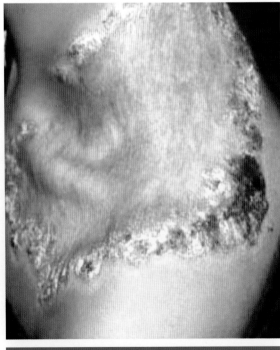

Lupus Vulgaris

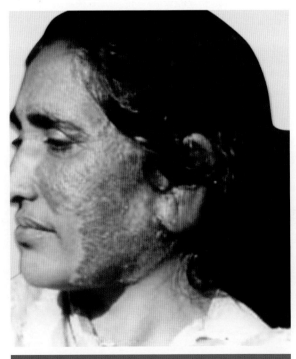

Lupus Vulgaris

CUTANEOUS TUBERCULOSIS

The common presentations of cutaneous tuberculosis are:

- Lupus vulgaris
- Scrofuloderma
- Tuberculus gumma
- Tuberculosis verrucosa cutis.

LUPUS VULGARIS

It is a slowly progressive, chronic tuberculosis of skin affecting people with a good immunity, and is characterized by the formation of caseous nodules. *Mycobacterium tuberculosis* gains access to the skin by direct inoculation, extension from underlying tuberculous glands or joints, lymphatic spread and hematogenously (rare). Tubercles are seen in upper dermis, composed of a focus of epithelioid cells with interspersed Langhans' giant cells and a peripheral rim of lymphocytes. There is a variable amount of perivascular infiltrate. Center of tubercle may undergo caseation necrosis or even calcify and ultimately fibrosis occurs. Initial lesion is a dusky red plaque which on diascopy (pressure with a glass slide), shows discrete, small, translucent nodules. These nodules are areas of caseation and due to their softness, can be penetrated by match stick. They are called "apple jelly" nodules because of their resemblance to it. Plaque spreads peripherally, with or without ulceration but with scarring. Destruction of underlying cartilage and mucosa can occur. Nose, eyelids, ears and mouth are usually affected. In long standing cases, squamous cell carcinoma may develop. Differential diagnosis includes psoriasis, sarcoidosis, discoid lupus erythematosus, leprosy, tertiary syphilis and leishmaniasis.

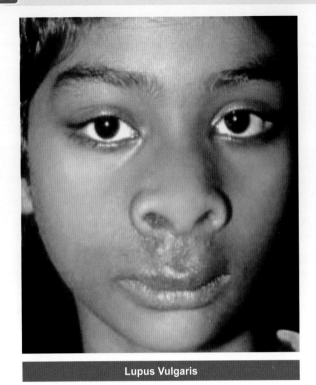

Lupus Vulgaris

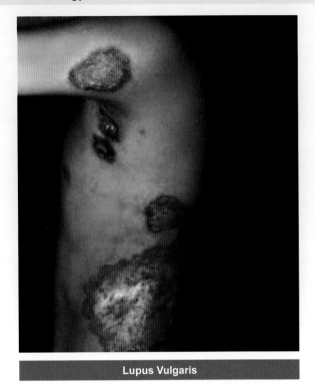

Lupus Vulgaris

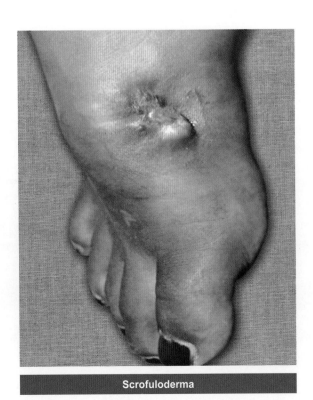

Scrofuloderma

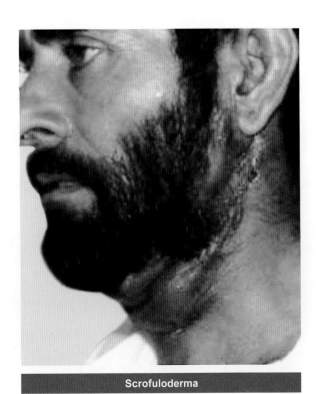

Scrofuloderma

SCROFULODERMA

Tuberculosis cutis colliquativa is the other name for this tuberculous infection. It arises as a direct extension from an underlying tuberculous focus, e.g. lymph node, bone or joint. Initial lesion is a bluish-red nodule which breaks down to form undermined ulcers and fistulae. Edges are undermined, inverted, with dissecting subcutaneous pockets alternating with soft, fluctuating infiltrates and bridging scars. Usually occurs in the parotid, submandibular and supraclavicular regions; lateral neck.

Diagnosis can be made by clinical findings, tuberculin skin testing and dermatopathology, confirmed by isolation of *M. tuberculosis* on culture or by PCR. The course of cutaneous tuberculosis is quite variable, and it depends upon the age of the patient and his/ her immune status, type of cutaneous infection, amount of inoculum, extent of extracutaneous involvement and therapy.

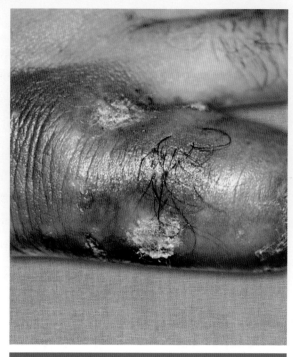

Scrofuloderma

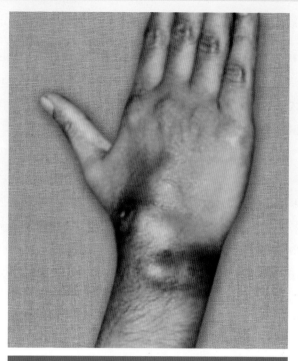

Tuberculous Gumma

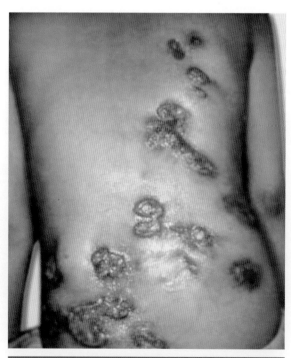

Tuberculous Gumma

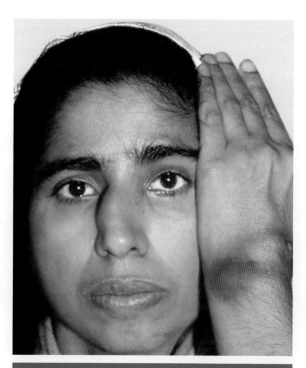

Tuberculous Gumma

TUBERCULOUS GUMMA

It is a rare form (1–2%) of cutaneous tuberculosis caused by hematogenous dissemination. "Metastatic tuberculous abscess" and "Metastatic tuberculous ulcer" are the synonyms of this condition. It is characterized histologically by the widespread caseation necrosis. It is the result of a hematogenous dissemination of tuberculous organisms from a primary lesion, leading to nodules which are erythematous, non-tender and firm in consistency. Later on, these nodules ulcerate, forming sinuses. Usual clinical presentation is either a fluctuant swelling or a firm subcutaneous nodule. In most of the cases, extremities are mainly affected as compared to the trunk. The skin slowly breaks down to give rise to an undermined ulcer/ sinuses. Rarely, secondary lesions may be seen, especially along the draining lymphatics. Lesions may be multiple in malnourished children. Diagnosis is confirmed by culture. Clinically, it is difficult to differentiate from atypical mycobacterial infection and subcutaneous fungal infections, syphilitic gumma and pyoderma gangrenosum. It should be confirmed by histopathology and culture.

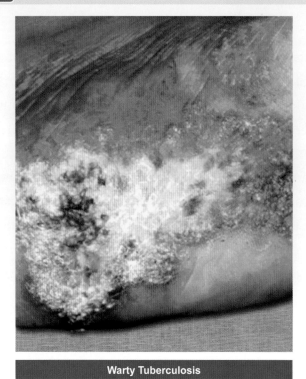

Warty Tuberculosis

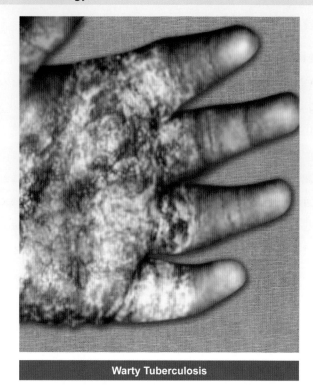

Warty Tuberculosis

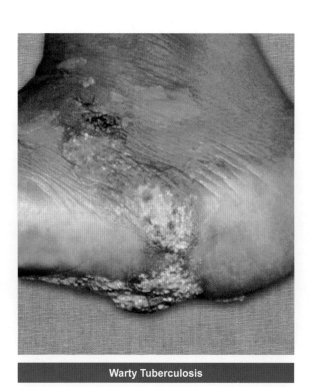

Warty Tuberculosis

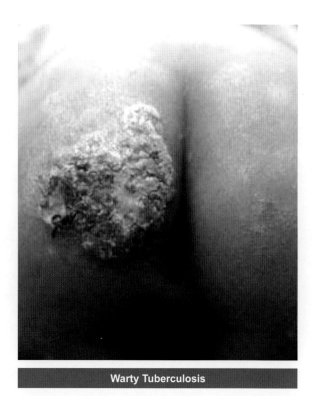

Warty Tuberculosis

WARTY TUBERCULOSIS (TUBERCULOSIS VERRUCOSA CUTIS)

It is a slow growing, verrucous type of tuberculosis, affecting the skin of an already infected person, with a good immunity. Infection can occur due to occupational exposure as seen in butchers, physicians, pathologists and postmortem attendants. In children and young adults, buttocks and legs may be affected by sitting and playing in contaminated streets. Initial lesion is a small, symptomless, purplish-red, indurated warty papule. It extends peripherally in a serpiginous fashion. Center may clear forming a scar or entire lesion may transform into a big warty mass. At times, crusting, exudation or pus may be seen. Differential diagnosis includes lichen planus hypertrophicus, tertiary syphilis, iodo- and bromoderma.

Treatment

Health of the patient should be improved by better nutrition and healthy environment. Intercurrent infection should be treated and any underlying disease, e.g. diabetes mellitus should be managed properly. In drug therapy, same principles are involved in treating cutaneous tuberculosis as that of any other organ. A combination of drugs should be used, keeping in mind the sensitivity and resistance of the *Mycobacterium tuberculosis* in a given area. The drugs and their daily dosages are: Rifampicin 450–600 mg, INH 300 mg, Ethambutol 0.7-I g, Pyrazinamide 1.5-2 g. Treatment is usually carried out with four drugs for 2 months and then two drugs for a total of 6 to 12 months.

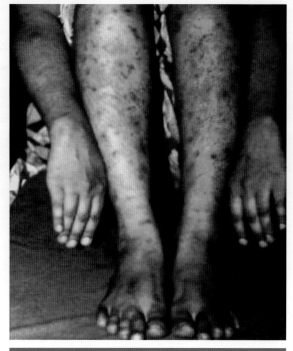

Papulonecrotic Tuberculide

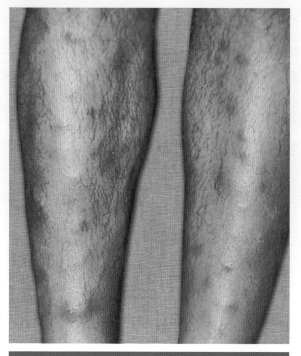

Papulonecrotic Tuberculide

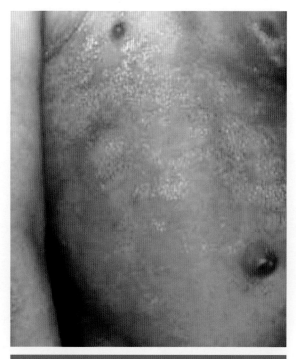

Lichen Scrofulosorum

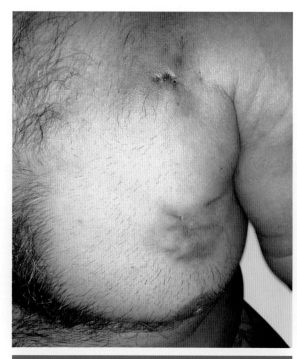

Swimming Pool Granuloma

TUBERCULIDES

These include skin lesions of various types in patients with a tuberculous focus elsewhere in the body. Tubercle bacillus cannot be isolated from the skin.

Papulonecrotic Tuberculide

It is a condition in which there is a crop of dusky-red necrotizing papules healing spontaneously to leave pigmented scars. Commonly affects hands, feet, arms, elbows, shoulders, legs and face. Fresh eruptions may continue to appear for months or years.

Lichen Scrofulosorum

It is common in young children or adolescents. Minute, skin colored or red, grouped, lichenoid papules appear, giving rise to a permanent goose skin appearance. Papules may be covered by small scales or spines, or occasionally pustules. Eruption persists for months and then involutes without scarring.

MYCOBACTERIUM MARINUM

Mycobacterium marinum is an atypical mycobacterial infection which is frequently noticed in swimmers. The natural habitat is unreplenished, heated up water in temperate climates (swimming pools, aquaria, rivers and beaches). The vectors are fresh and salt water fish, snails, shellfish and water flees. Cutaneous lesions appear after 2–3 weeks up to 9 months. The sites of involvement are cooler extremities, i.e. hands, arms, shoulders. It can start as a single nodule or pustule which changes into ulcer, abscess and sinuses. The lesions may be multiple in sporotrichoid pattern. It is usually seen in immunocompromized patients. Antibiotics like sulphamethoxazole + trimethoprim, minocycline, doxycycline, rifampicin + ethambutol, clarithromycim, levofloxacin or amikacin can be given for a duration of 14 weeks or longer.

SEXUALLY TRANSMITTED DISEASES

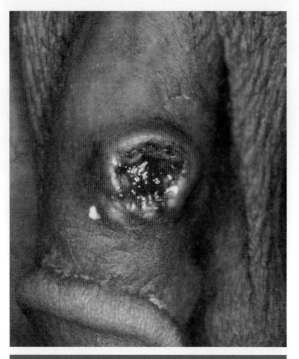

Syphilitic Chancre

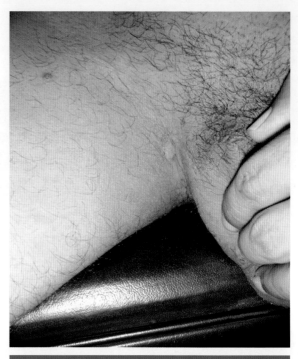

Syphilitic Chancre

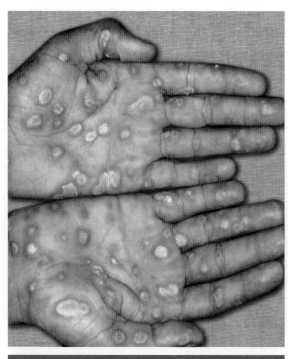

Secondary Syphilis

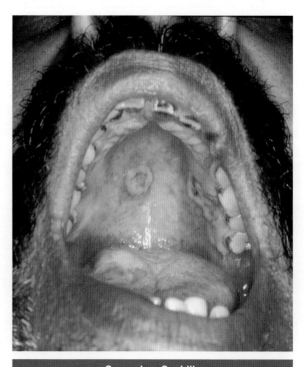

Secondary Syphilis

SYPHILIS

It is a chronic infection caused by a spirochaete called Treponema pallidum, capable of penetrating skin and mucosa and is principally acquired by sexual contact. Occasionally, it is caused by handling infected material or blood transfusion. There is also a congenital form. It is customary to divide acquired syphilis into three stages, i.e. primary, secondary and tertiary.

Primary Syphilis is characterized by the formation of a chancre 10–30 days after the infection associated with regional lymphadenopathy. Chancre is typically a painless indurated ulcer with sharp margins and a smooth glazed surface. In men, it is located on coronal sulcus, glans penis, shaft of penis or the inner surface of prepuce and in women on vulva, vagina or cervix uteri. Extragenital chancre occurs on lips, tongue, tonsils, eyelids, fingers, nipples or perianal region. It heals without treatment in 3–8 weeks, leaving a thin atrophic scar. Differential diagnosis includes chancroid, scabies, herpes genitalis, lichen planus, carcinoma of penis, drug eruptions, lymphogranuloma venereum and traumatic ulcer. Diagnosis is confirmed by dark ground microscopic examination of serum taken from the chancre for the presence of treponema. Serological tests for syphilis, e.g. VDRL, are useless at this stage.

Secondary Syphilis is characterized by the appearance, 6–8 weeks after the primary chancre, of generalized skin eruptions (syphilides) which occur as recurrent and polymorphic lesions (macular, papular or pustular), never bullous or itchy as a rule. Macular syphilides are the first to appear, affecting the trunk, face, limbs, and soles. Lesions are rose colored hence called roseola and on fading leave depigmentation particularly around the neck (necklace of Venus). Papular eruption is deeply infiltrated and dull red in color which may assume annular or circinate shape.

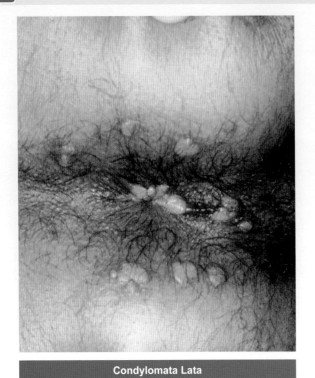

Condylomata Lata

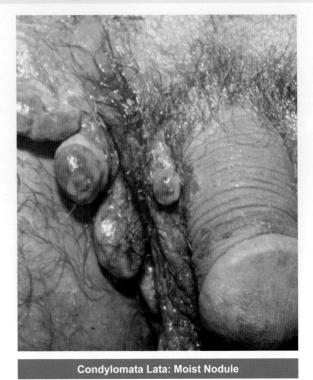

Condylomata Lata: Moist Nodule

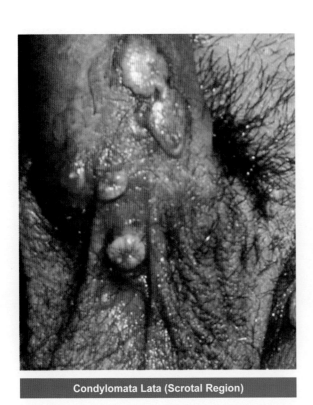

Condylomata Lata (Scrotal Region)

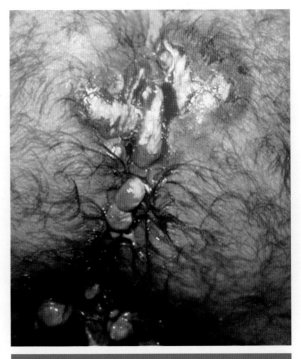

Condylomata Lata (Anal Region): Multiple Moist Nodules

Mucosal lesions of secondary syphilis include snail track ulcers or mucos patches in the mouth. There are hypertrophic, moist, soggy plaques at muco-cutaneons junctions called condylomata lata. Lymphadenopathy is generalized, discrete, painless and mobile. Diagnostically most important glands are those of posterior triangle of neck, occipital, auricular, axillary and supratrochlear region. Constitutional symptoms are headache, malaise, low grade pyrexia, hoarseness, anemia and splenomegaly.

Miscellaneous symptoms include alopecia which may be patchy (moth-eaten type) or diffuse, paronychia, iridocyclitis, periostitis and rarely arthritis. Serological tests for syphilis are positive in 100% cases. Differential diagnosis includes pityriasis rosea, fungal infection, seborrheic dermatitis, psoriasis and drug eruptions.

Treatment

Intramuscular penicillin is still the mainstay of treatment in all forms of the disease. Procaine penicillin 600,000 units are given daily for 10–14 days, or Procaine penicillin G in oil with 2% aluminum monostearate (PAM) 4.8 mega units is administered, or benzathine penicillin in a single dose of 2.4 mega units, is the treatment given in early syphilis. In those who are sensitive to penicillin, erythromycin 500 mg four times a day for 2 weeks or tetracycline 750 mg four times a day for 2 weeks, can be given. In syphilis of more than one year duration, a longer treatment is required, e.g. weekly injections of 2.4 mega units of benzathine penicillin for 3 weeks. Similarly, erythromycin and tetracycline are given for one month in a dose of 500 mg QID. In congenital syphilis, only one dose of benzathine penicillin 50,000 units per kg body weight is given. Pregnant ladies with syphilis should be treated early to prevent or minimize fetal involvement.

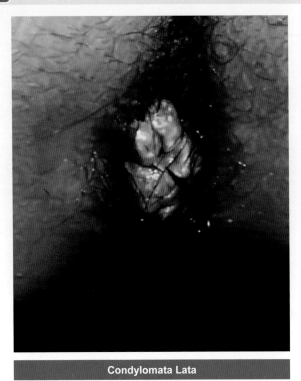

Condylomata Lata

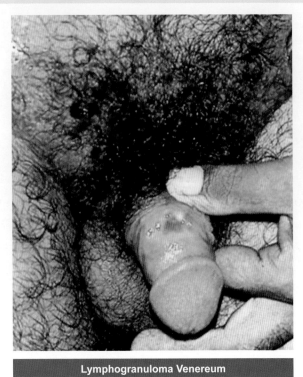

Lymphogranuloma Venereum

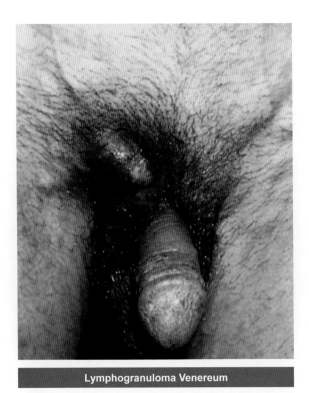

Lymphogranuloma Venereum

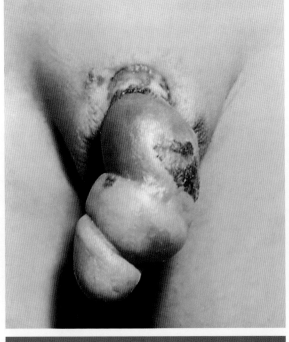

Saxophone Penis

LYMPHOGRANULOMA VENEREUM

It is a chronic infection characterized by constitutional symptoms and matted inguinal lymphadenopathy, i.e. inguinal buboes which ulcerate. The causative agent is *Chlamydia trachomatis*. Incubation period is 3–20 days. Lymphadenopathy, above and below the inguinal ligament, results in the groove sign. Primary rectal involvement may lead to stricture formation. Elephantiasis of the female genitalia with chronic ulceration and scarring of vulva (esthiomene) may occur. Scarring and lymphedema in males may result in saxophone penis. Cutaneous manifestations include erythema multiforme, erythema nodosum, photosensitivity and scarlatiniform eruption. Pyrexia, weight loss, anemia, arthritis, colitis, glossitis, conjunctivitis, meningitis and pneumonia are other systemic manifestations. Complement fixation test becomes positive after four weeks. Treatment consists of doxycycline 100 mg two times daily or erythromycin 500 mg QID for 3 weeks. Incision and drainage or needle aspiration may be required to treat the abscesses. In complicated cases, help of a surgeon may be needed for colostomy for rectal obstruction, dilatation of the rectal stricture, or repair of rectovaginal fistulae.

LEPROSY

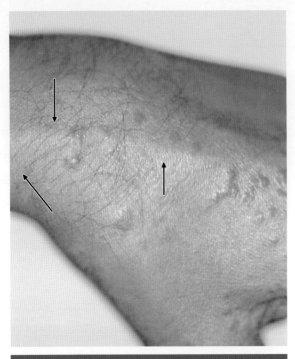

Leprosy

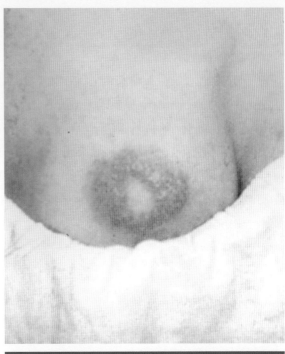

Borderline Leprosy: Saucer-shaped Erythematous
Scaly Plaque

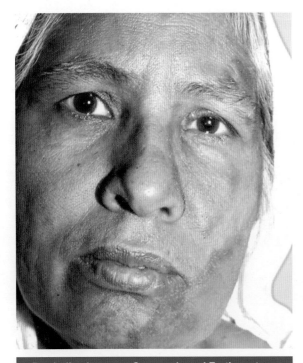

Borderline Leprosy: Saucer-shaped Erythematous
Plaque

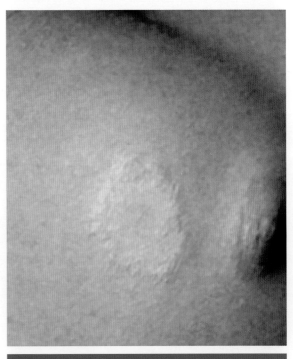

Borderline Leprosy

Leprosy is a contagious infection, which runs a chronic course. Primary affected organs are the peripheral nerves while skin and mucous membranes of the mouth and upper respiratory tract are secondarily involved, along with the eyes, bones, reticuloendothelial system and testes. The causative agent is *Mycobacterium leprae* (discovered by Hansen in 1873). Spread depends upon prolonged contact and high genetic susceptibility. There are four types depending upon immunity against the *Mycobacterium leprae*.

BORDERLINE LEPROSY

This variety occupies middle position between tuberculoid and lepromatous types. Depending upon the degree of immunity, it may be borderline tuberculoid (BT), mid-borderline (BB) or borderline lepromatous (BL). Accordingly, BT gives a positive lepromin test while it is negative in BL. Clinical features depend upon the type. Nerves and skin are the only tissues directly involved. Skin lesions consist of erythematous macules and plaques. Annular lesions are common with a band of well-defined erythema surrounding a hypopigmented center.

INDETERMINATE LEPROSY

It is a type with transitional immune status. Lepromin test is unpredictable. Nerves and skin are involved. Cutaneous lesions comprise of asymmetrical, nondescript macules. Diagnostic tests include skin smear for *M. leprae*, histopathology of a biopsy specimen from skin or nerve and Lepromin test. Differential diagnosis includes pityriasis alba, lupus vulgaris, discoid lupus erythematosus, drug eruption, guttate psoriasis, granuloma annulare and sarcoidosis.

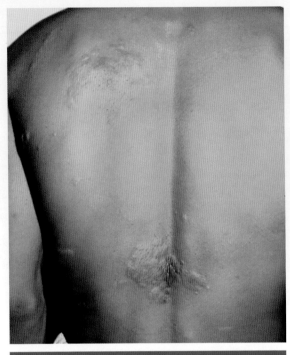

Borderline Leprosy

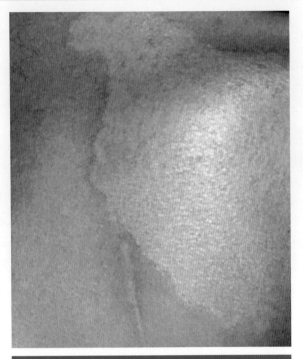

Tuberculoid Leprosy: Hypopigmented well defined dry plaque

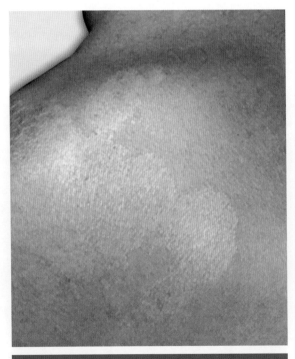

Tuberculoid Leprosy

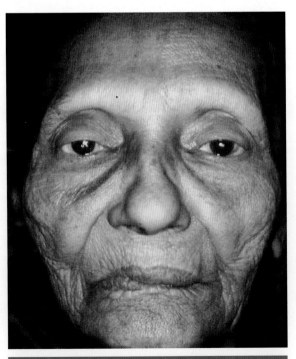

Madarosis

TUBERCULOID LEPROSY

The tissues directly affected are only nerves and skin. Cutaneous lesions consist of erythematous, pigmented or hypopigmented macules which are dry, anesthetic and anhidrotic. Edges are raised and well-defined. Nerves are thickened with associated anesthesia and muscle weakness. Ulnar, peroneal and greater auricular nerves are palpably thickened. Eye damage is due to involvement of trigeminal and facial nerves. There is resorption of distal bones of hands and feet with associated trophic ulceration of skin. In this type, lepromin test is positive (denoting high immunity). Bacilli are few in number.

LEPROMATOUS LEPROSY

Cutaneous changes are the first to appear, showing bilaterally symmetrical eruption of slightly hypopigmented macules, papules, plaques and nodules. There is predilection for face, limbs and buttocks. Hair growth and sensation remain intact. Later changes include ulceration of nasal and buccal mucosa and other parts of the body, diffuse thickening of skin (leonine facies), ophthalmic damage, testicular atrophy, gynecomastia, absorption of bone and late stage peripheral nerve damage. In this type, lepromin test is negative (denoting no immunity). Bacilli are found in large numbers. Acute reactions may follow treatment particularly with dapsone. Such reactions, seen in lepromatous leprosy, may be precipitated by stress, intercurrent infection, pregnancy or injury. Either the existing lesions may become prominent (Type I) or erythema nodosum leprosum (Type II) may be seen.

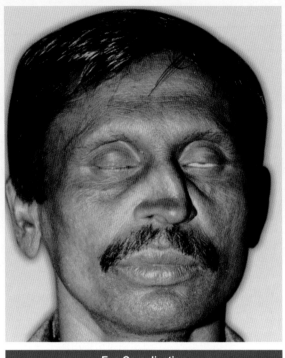

Eye Complication

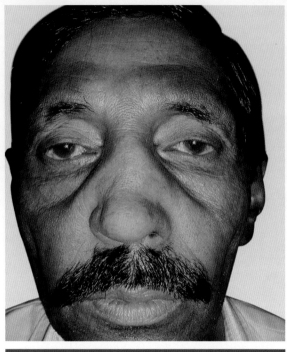

Eye Complication

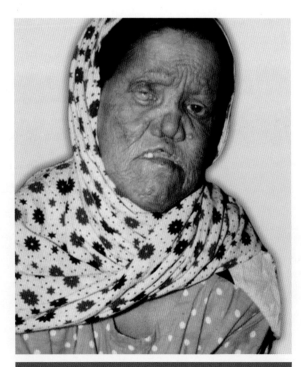

Leonine Facies, Collapsed Nose and Eye Involvement

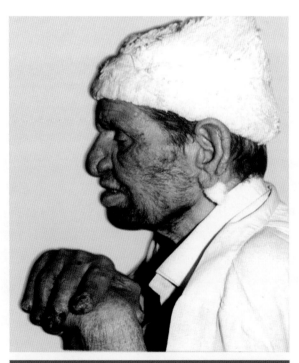

Leonine Facies, Collapsed Nose and Eczematous Changes

COMPLICATIONS

Help of plastic surgeon, orthopedic surgeon and physiotherapist is sometimes required for disfiguring lesions and paralyzed muscles, etc.

PREVENTION

Advise the patient to elevate the living standards and improve public health education.

TREATMENT

Treatment is done mainly on outpatient basis. Hospitalization is necessary only for patients with reactions, side effects of drugs or for surgical treatment of complications. With emergence of resistance against drugs, e.g. dapsone, rifampicin, clofazimine and ethionamide, WHO has recommended multiple drug treatment (MDT). Number of drugs used and length of treatment varies according to the type of leprosy as follows:

Multibacillary leprosy (Lepromatous and BL): Rifampicin 600 mg once a month (supervised) or 50 mg daily (unsupervised), Dapsone 100mg daily (unsupervised), Clofazimine 50 mg daily (unsupervised) or 300mg monthly supervised, treatment should be continued for one year for patients with a bacillary index (BI) of less than +3 and two years for BI above +4 and surveillance for five years afterwards.

Paucibacillary leprosy (Tuberculoid and BT): Rifampicin 600 mg once a month (supervised), Dapsone 100 mg daily (unsupervised), treatment should be continued for six months and surveillance for further two years.

TREATMENT OF REACTIONS

Anti-leprosy drug therapy is maintained in full dosage. Type I reaction requires 40–80 mg prednisolone daily with gradual reduction over 4–9 months. Type II reactions are treated with bed rest, analgesics and prednisolone 60 mg daily with rapid tapering over a month. Alternatively, thalidomide 100 mg thrice daily, or clofazimine 300 mg daily, may be used. Pain in the motor nerves can be relieved by intraneural injection of a mixture of hyaluronidase 1500 units, 1 ml of 2% lignocaine and 1 ml of hydrocortisone suspension (25 mg/ml) given with a size 14 needle. Iridocyclitis is treated with 1% hydrocortisone eye drops and mydriatics, e.g. 1% atropine.

SCABIES

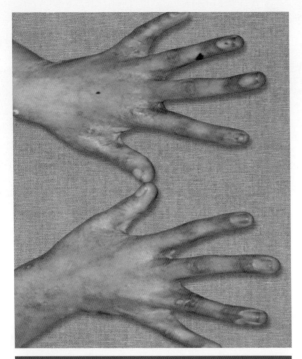

Scabies Burrows

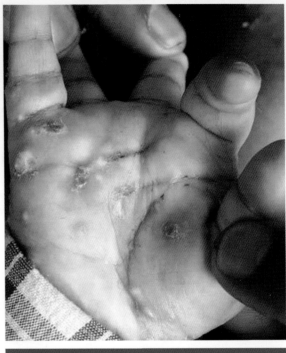

Scabies (Pusular Lesions)

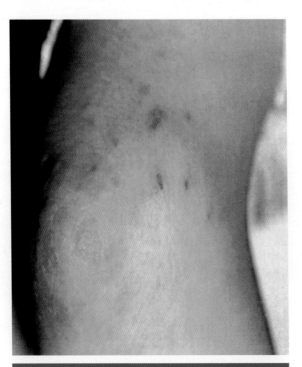

Scabies (Burrows on elbow)

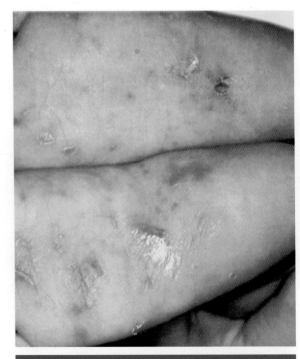

Scabies Burrows

SCABIES

Scabies is a contagious parasitic disorder often occurring in epidemics. It is caused by a minute mite, i.e. Sarcoptes (Acarus) scabiei. Fertilized females burrow into the skin laying eggs which after hatching moult three times to become adults. Cycle is repeated every 14–17 days. The disease affects all ages and both sexes. Severe itching occurs, usually nocturnal in character. More than one family member is often affected by sleeping together. Latent period before itching develops is 2–6 weeks. Characteristic lesions are burrows which are grayish linear, C-shaped or S-shaped, slightly raised lesions seen in typical sites, e.g. interdigital clefts, ulnar border of hands, wrists, elbows, axillae, umbilicus, buttocks, penis, breasts and nipples. Palms and soles of feet are affected in infants. Face is usually not affected except in children. Penile lesions look like blind boils. Discrete papules, vesicles and pustules appear secondarily and dominate the clinical picture. Less commonly, Norwegian (crusted) scabies, seen in immunocompromised patients, is characterized by heavy scaling and crusting harbouring numerous mites. Itching may not be pronounced. Complications include secondary infection, e.g. impetigo, boils and ecthyma, eczematization particularly in infants and persistent itchy post-scabetic nodules. Diagnosis is confirmed by scraping a burrow with a scalpel, putting a small amount of KOH 10% solution and finally looking under the microscope for the acarus or the eggs. Nocturnal itching and involvement of more than one family members is very suggestive.

Treatment

There should be treatment of the patient and all other inmates of the house whether itching or not. The topical preparation should be applied on whole body below collar line (entire body in infants). Laundering of clothes should be done and no special disinfection is required. Scabies should be treated first and complications later. Medicaments used are: 25% benzyl benzoate emulsion (12.5% for children below seven), 1% gamma benzene hexachloride cream and lotion, 10% sulphur ointment (2.5% for infants), 25% monosulfiram lotion, 10% crotamiton cream, 0.5% malathion lotion, 5% permethrin cream and lotion. Single oral dose of Ivermectin, 200 mg/ kg can be given and may be repeated weekly twice or thrice.

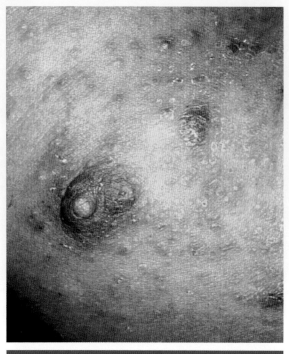

Scabies (Lesion on Breast)

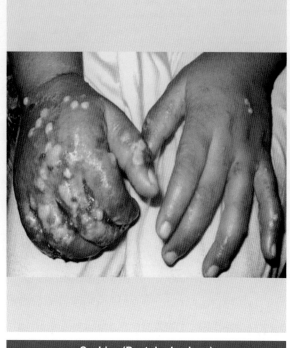

Scabies (Pustular Lesions)

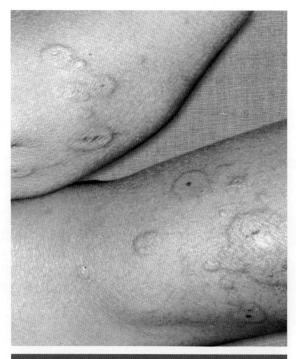

Papular Urticaria

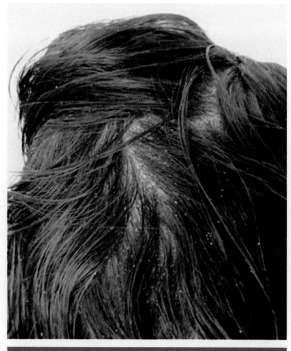

Pediculosis Capitis

PEDICULOSIS CAPITIS (HEAD LOUSE)

It is almost confined to scalp but rarely invades beard or exceptionally other hairy areas. Density of population is usually highest in the occipital and preauricular regions. Infestation occurs by combs and shared head gear. Long hair and infrequent washing increase susceptibility. Women and children are commonly affected. Itching is most marked around the occipital region and sides of scalp. Secondary infection with suboccipital adenitis is common and may be the presenting complaint. Nits on the occipital region resemble scales. Hair may be matted together with pus, producing foul odour. Diagnosis is confirmed by the presence of lice or nits.

Treatment

1% gamma benzene hexachloride cream and lotion, 5% permethrin cream and lotion, 0.5% carbaryl lotion, 0.5% malathion lotion.

PAPULAR URTICARIA (LICHEN URTICATUS)

It is an eruption of recurrent pruritic papules, usually grouped and mostly seasonal, typically occurring in young children due to insect bites. Examples of offending insects include fleas, bed bugs, mosquitoes, midges and lice. Papular urticaria is uncommon before the age of two because of lack of sensitivity and after the age of seven due to development of hyposensitization. There are irritable weals, often in clusters, surmounted by papules or occasionally bullae. Recurrent crops lasting two to ten days leave pigmentation. Distribution depends upon the type of insect. Airborne insects often bite on the exposed parts like hands, face, arms, neck and lower legs. Fleas and bed bugs produce lesions mainly on the trunk. Secondary infection is common.

Treatment

Prevention against insects is most important. Family pets like dogs or cats, or bird's nests may be the source. Spraying of insecticides inside the house is useful. Once the lesions have appeared, 1% phenol or 1% menthol in calamine lotion will be soothing. Oral antihistamines are also useful.

LEISHMANIASIS

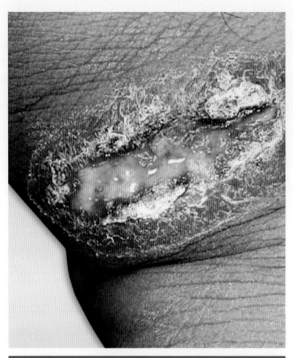

Cutaneous Leishmaniasis

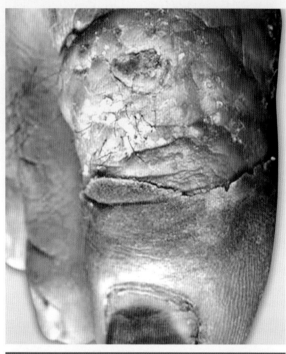

Cutaneous Leishmaniasis

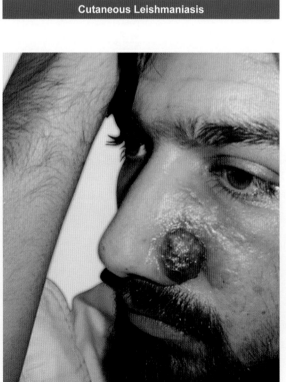

Cutaneous Leishmaniasis

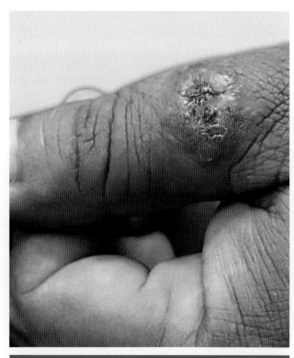

Cutaneous Leishmaniasis

CUTANEOUS LEISHMANIASIS

It is also called Lahore sore, Quetta boil, Delhi boil, Mughal sore and oriental sore. There are various species of Leishmania, e.g. *L. tropica*, *L. major*, *L. aethiopica* and *L. infantum*. Cutaneous leishmaniasis is transmitted by sandflies, e.g. Phlebotomus papatasii and Phlebotomus sergenti in Pakistan. L. major, a zoonosis, is commonly seen in gerbils while *L. tropica* is primarily a disease of human beings. Two acute forms (wet and dry) and a chronic form (recidivans) are seen.

a. **Wet (Rural):** It is caused by *L. major*. Incubation period is less than two months. There are red nodules at the site of inoculation which ulcerate while increasing in size. Multiple, small secondary nodules may appear surrounding the original lesion and along lymphatics (skip lesions) and healing occurs in 2-6 months with scarring.

b. **Dry (Urban):** It is caused by *L. tropica*. There is a longer incubation period of more than two months. Small brownish nodule enlarges into a plaque. Ulceration occurs followed by crusting. Secondary nodules are commonly seen. Healing occurs after 8–12 months with scarring.

c. **Recidivans (Lupoid):** It is due to a peculiar host reaction but not to any particular strain of *L. tropica*. Brown red papules appear in the near vicinity of an old scar of leishmaniasis. A plaque is formed by the coalescence of papules which resembles lupus vulgaris. This is very chronic in nature lasting many years. Demonstration of the parasite is from a scraping taken from the edge of the ulcer. Culture can be done for *L. tropica* (on NNN medium). Leishmanin test becomes positive within three months. Differential diagnosis includes lupus vulgaris, tertiary syphilis and desert sore.

Treatment

Sodium stibogluconate (Pentostam) 20 mg/kg intramuscular daily (maximum 850 mg) for 10–20 days. Meglumine antimoniate (Glucantime) 60 mg/kg body weight intramuscular daily (maximum 850 mg) for 10–14 days. Cryotherapy e.g. liquid nitrogen and CO_2 snow can be used locally. Prophylaxis is done by sandfly control measures and immunization with cultures of *L. tropica*.

Chapter 2

BULLOUS DISORDERS

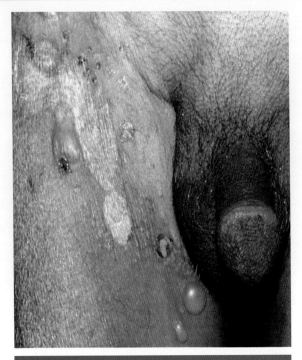

Pemphigus Vulgaris

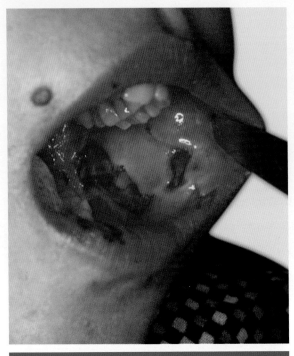

Pemphigus Vulgaris

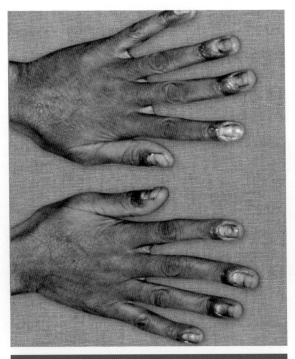

Pemphigus Vulgaris with Paronychia

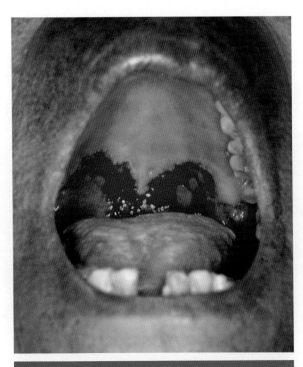

Pemphigus Vulgaris

PEMPHIGUS VULGARIS

It is an autoimmune, bullous disorder affecting the skin and mucous membranes. The blisters are intraepithelial, caused by the circulating autoantibodies which are directed against the keratinocyte desmosomal protein desmoglein-3. Oral mucous membrane is involved in almost all cases. The patients may present with irregular painful buccal, gingival or palatine erosions, which are slow to heal. There may be a downward spread involving the larynx, leading to hoarseness. In more than 50% cases of pemphigus vulgaris occurring in younger age groups, oral involvement is the first symptom. Additional mucosal surfaces which can be involved, like the conjunctiva, esophagus, nasal mucosa, labia, vagina, cervix, penis, urethra and anus. The blister is flaccid and filled with a clear fluid, arising on a healthy or erythematous skin. Bullae rupture easily, giving rise to painful erosions. Nails may be affected in the form of acute or chronic paronychia or subungual hematomas. Nail dystrophies may also be seen affecting one or several nails. When the skin folds are affected, the lesions take the form of verrucous granulations. The treatment consists of corticosteroids. Steroid-sparing immunosuppressants like mycophenolate mofetil and azathioprine should be considered early. Cyclophosphamide, rituximab and intravenous immunoglobulins have also proven to be useful adjuncts.

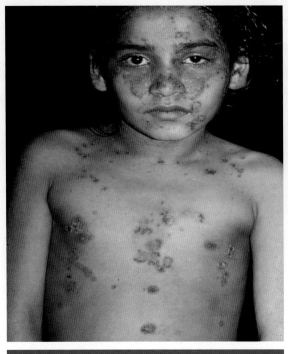

Pemphigus Foliaceus

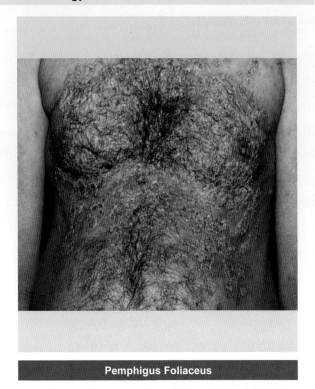

Pemphigus Foliaceus

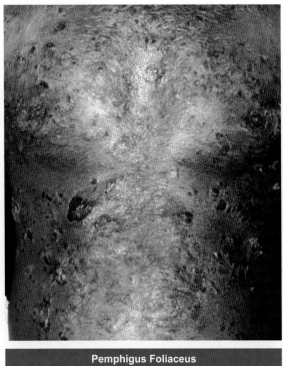

Pemphigus Foliaceus

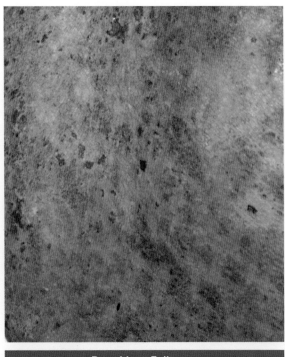

Pemphigus Foliaceus

PEMPHIGUS FOLIACEUS

It is a benign type of pemphigus, characterized by the formation of superficial intraepithelial blisters. Pathognomonic antibodies are directed against desmoglein-1 of the desmosome. The blisters are rarely seen in this disease. They are very fragile due to their superficial location, hence they rupture leaving behind a mild scaling. When, however, they are present, a tangential pressure on the perilesional skin leads to extension of bullae as does a vertical pressure on its roof. The former is known as Nikolsky's sign and the latter as bulla spreading sign. P. foliaceus usually involves the seborrheic areas and runs a chronic course, with occasional involvement of the mucous membranes. It is divided into six types: pemphigus erythematosus, pemphigus herpetiformis, endemic pemphigus foliaceus, endemic pemphigus foliaceus with antigenic reactivity characteristic of paraneoplastic pemphigus (but with no neoplasm), immunoglobulin A (IgA) pemphigus foliaceus and drug-induced pemphigus foliaceus. Treatment consists of systemic steroids in combination with immunosuppressants. Some cases require the anti-CD20 monoclonal antibody, rituximab. Intravenous immunoglobulin may also be used due to its minimizing effects on circulating antibodies. Simultaneous administration of a cytotoxic drug may also be beneficial.

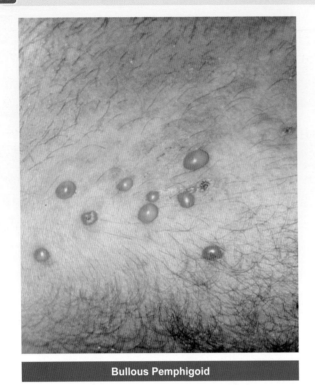

Bullous Pemphigoid

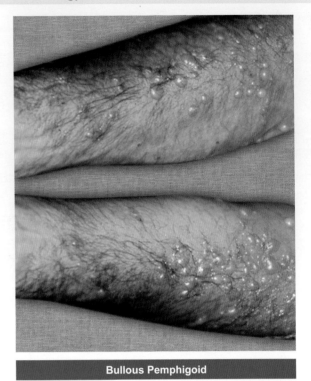

Bullous Pemphigoid

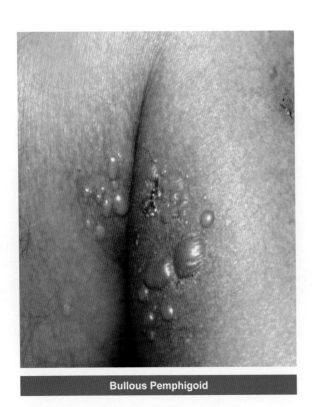

Bullous Pemphigoid

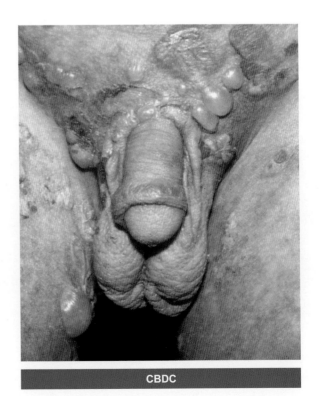

CBDC

BULLOUS PEMPHIGOID

It is an inflammatory, chronic, subepidermal bullous disorder. It may manifest with several distinct clinical presentations as: ***a generalized bullous form***, the commonest variety, in which tense blisters are formed anywhere on the body, with flexural areas being the favored sites; ***vesicular form***, appears as small, tense bullae on an erythematous base, often arranged in groups; ***vegetative form***, presents with verrucous plaques in the flexural areas of the body, such as the axillae, groin and inframammary areas; ***generalized erythrodermic form***, mimicks psoriasis, eczema especially atopic dermatitis, or exfoliative dermatitis caused by other skin conditions; ***urticarial form***, is characterized by persistent weals which can later on turn into bullous lesions; ***nodular form***, the clinical features resemble with those of prurigo nodularis, blisters arise on the normal or nodular lesions; ***acral form***, is bullous pemphigoid occurring in childhood, sometimes following vaccination, blisters mainly affecting the face, palms and soles; ***infant form***, the blisters tend to occur frequently on the palms, soles and face, rarely on the genital areas; 60% of these cases have generalized bullae. The main goal of treatment is to reduce the formation of blisters, early healing and determine the minimal dose of drug necessary to control the disease. Commonly used drugs are anti-inflammatory agents, such as steroids, tetracyclines or dapsone and immunosuppressants like azathioprine, mycophenolate mofetil, methotrexate and cyclophosphamide.

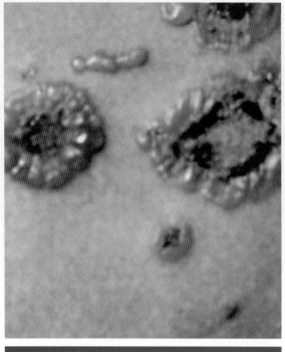

CBDC, Rosette Lesions, Cluster of Jewels

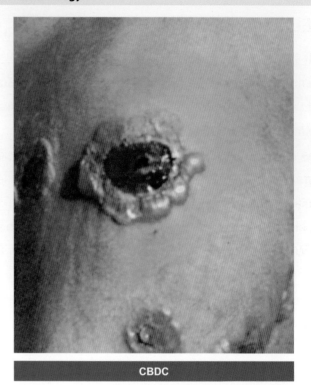

CBDC

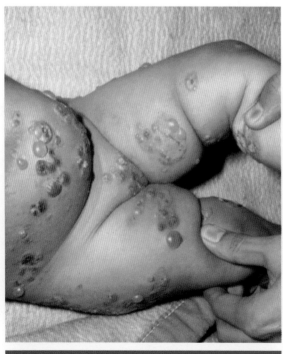

Chronic Bullous Disease of Childhood

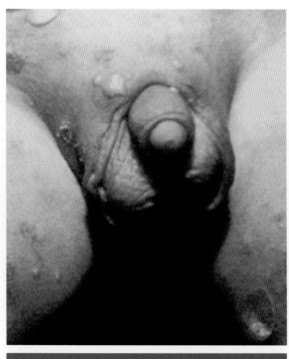

CBDC

LINEAR IMMUNOGLOBULIN A (IGA) DERMATOSIS

It is a subepidermal blistering disorder. The cause may be unknown or it may be produced by drugs. Patients of any age can be affected, the disease occurring in children is called ***chronic bullous dermatosis of childhood***. Sometimes, the disease presents with a prolonged prodromal period of pruritus or burning. Those with eye involvement may present with grittiness, pain, or discharge. Blisters may be chronic, or they may have an acute onset, especially in drug-induced cases. In drug-induced cases of linear IgA dermatosis, the latent period may be as long as 1–13 days after taking the drug (vancomycin). The classical presentation is a clear and/or hemorrhagic, round or oval blister on a normal, or erythematous skin. Other manifestations may be blanching macules and papules, erythematous plaques, or targetoid EM-like lesions.

Blisters can be solitary or arranged in a grouped (herpetiform) manner, which is known as the ***cluster of jewels sign***. Otherwise, vesico-bullous lesions may arise at the periphery of annular or circinate lesions, this condition has been called ***string of beads sign***. In children, the lesions are classically localized to the lower abdomen and anogenital areas. Other areas such as the feet, hands, and face, especially the perioral area may also be involved. In adults, the most common sites affected are trunk and limbs. In both age groups, the lesions may be seen in a symmetrical or asymmetrical manner. Involvement of the extensor surfaces of elbows and knees like the dermatitis herpetiformis, is an infrequent finding. Crusts, excoriations, erosions, or ulcers may be found.

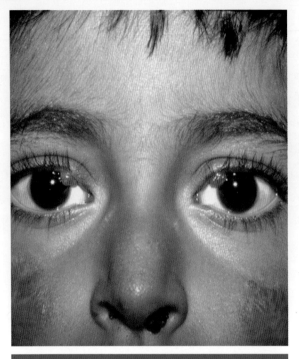

Shabbir's Syndrome

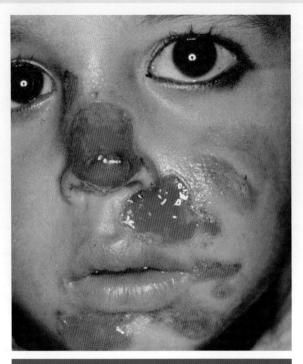

Shabbir's Syndrome

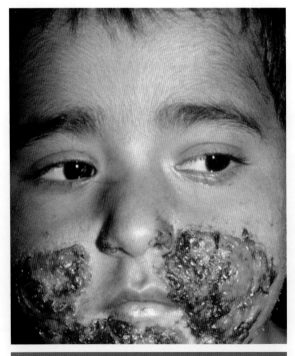

Shabbir's Syndrome, Crusted erosions involving the periorificial areas

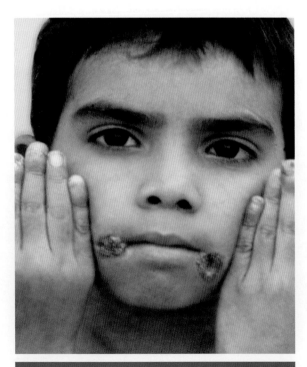

Shabbir's Syndrome

Oral involvement is common manifesting as blisters, erosions, ulcerations, erythematous areas, erosive cheilitis or desquamative gingivitis, and they may be seen before the skin lesions appear. The patients frequently complain of eye symptoms, like burning, grittiness, or discharge. Subconjunctival fibrosis, shrinkage of the fornices, symblepharon formation, and cicatricial entropion with trichiasis, are the findings which may be seen even in the absence of ocular complaints. Dapsone or sulphapyridine give good results within 48–72 hours.

SHABBIR'S SYNDROME

Shabbir's Syndrome, also known as **laryngo-onycho-cutaneous syndrome**, is a junctional type of epidermolysis bullosa with autosomal recessive inheritance. Epidermolysis bullosa (EB) is a disease complex classified as mechanobullous disorder, associated with skin erosions, blistering and/ or scarring of skin and mucous membranes as a result of mild mechanical trauma. This fragility results from abnormality of various components in the hemidesmosomes, the lamina lucida of the basement membrane zone or sublamina densa area. Accordingly, the disease is classified as EB simplex, junctional and dystrophica respectively, with the disease severity increasing in the same order. Shabbir's syndrome refers to involvement of the larynx, the nails and the skin. Hence, apart from vesicles and bullae on frictional sites, there may be hoarseness of voice and nail dystrophy or complete anonychia. Diagnosis requires electron microscopic examination of the perilesional biopsy specimen transported in glutaraldehyde.

Chapter **3**

DRUG REACTIONS

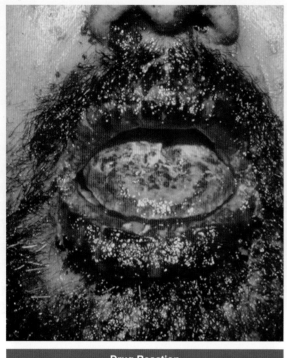

Drug Reaction

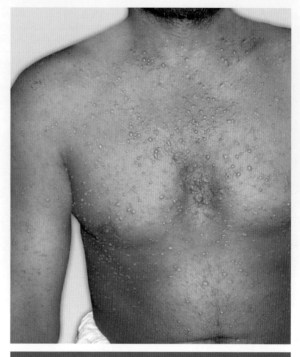

Drug Reaction

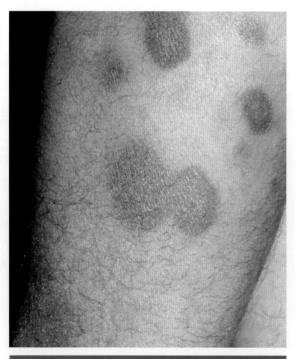

Erythema Multiforme

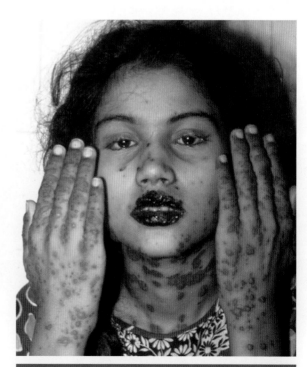

Stevens-Johnson Syndrome

Drug-induced cutaneous disorders frequently display a characteristic clinical morphology such as morbilliform exanthem, urticaria, hypersensitivity syndrome, pseudolymphoma, photosensitivity, pigmentary changes, acute generalized exanthematous pustulosis, lichenoid dermatitis, vasculitis, Stevens-Johnson syndrome, or fixed drug eruption (FDE).

ERYTHEMA MULTIFORME

Erythema multiforme (EM) is an acute, self-limited and sometimes recurring skin condition that is considered to be a type IV hypersensitivity reaction associated with certain infections, medications, and various other triggers. *Erythema multiforme minor* represents a localized eruption of the skin with minimal or no mucosal involvement. The papules evolve into pathognomonic target lesions or iris lesions that appear within a 72-hour period. More severe erosions of at least 2 mucosal surfaces are seen in *erythema multiforme major* and are characterized by hemorrhagic crusting of the lips (25%) and ulceration of the nonkeratinized mucosa. Occasionally, painful mucosal involvement may be extensive, with few or no skin lesions. Mucosal lesions usually heal without sequelae. The mucosal involvement in **Stevens-Johnson syndrome** is more severe and more extensive than that of erythema multiforme major. Generalized lymphadenopathy often accompanies erythema multiforme major. Erythema multiforme and Stevens-Johnson syndrome have different precipitating and clinical patterns and are generally recognized to be separate clinical entities. No specific laboratory tests are indicated to make the diagnosis of erythema multiforme (EM), which should be arrived at clinically. The most important treatment is usually symptomatic, including oral antihistamines, analgesics, local skin care, and soothing mouthwashes (e.g. oral rinsing with warm saline or a solution of diphenhydramine, xylocaine and kaopectate). Topical steroids may be considered. If a drug is suspected, it must be withdrawn as soon as possible. This includes all medications begun during the preceding 2 months. Infections should be appropriately treated after cultures. Prophylaxis for recurrence of herpes-associated erythema multiforme (HAEM) should be considered in patients with more than 5 attacks per year. Low-dose acyclovir (200 mg qid to 400 mg bid) can be effective for recurrence of HAEM, even in subclinical herpes simplex virus (HSV) infection. In children, 10 mg/kg/day may be considered.

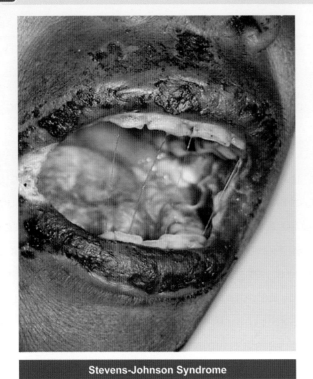

Stevens-Johnson Syndrome

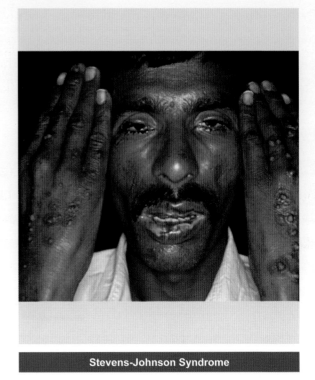

Stevens-Johnson Syndrome

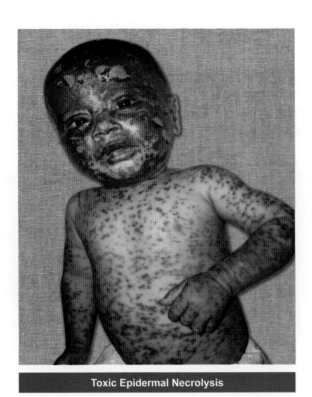

Toxic Epidermal Necrolysis

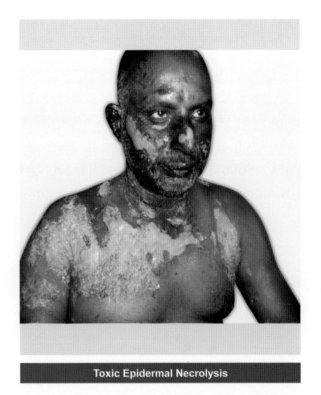

Toxic Epidermal Necrolysis

TOXIC EPIDERMAL NECROLYSIS

Toxic epidermal necrolysis (TEN), an acute disorder, is characterized by widespread erythematous macules and targetoid lesions; full-thickness epidermal necrosis, at least focally; and involvement of more than 30% of the cutaneous surface. Commonly, the mucous membranes are also involved. Nearly all cases of toxic epidermal necrolysis are induced by medications, and the mortality rate can approach 40%. Constitutional symptoms such as fever, cough, or sore throat, may appear 1–3 days prior to any cutaneous lesions. Patients may complain of a burning sensation in their eyes, photophobia, and a burning rash that begins symmetrically on the face and upper part of the torso. Delineation of a drug exposure timeline is essential, especially in the 1–3 weeks preceding the cutaneous eruption. The initial skin lesions of toxic epidermal necrolysis are poorly defined, erythematous macules with darker, purpuric centers. The lesions differ from classic target lesions of erythema multiforme by having only 2 zones of color: a central, dusky purpura or a central bulla, with a surrounding macular erythema. A classic target lesion has 3 zones of color: a central, dusky purpura or a central bulla; a surrounding pale, edematous zone; and an outer range of macular erythema.

Other findings in Stevens-Johnson syndrome/ toxic epidermal necrolysis include painful oral erosions causing severe crusting of the lips, increased salivation, and impaired alimentation. Lesions have been reported in the oropharynx, tracheobronchial tree, esophagus, gastrointestinal tract, genitalia, and anus. Involvement of the genitalia may lead to painful micturition. Intact expectorated cylindrical casts of bronchial epithelium have been reported; patients may develop a profuse, protein-rich diarrhea; internal involvement is not necessarily limited to patients with extensive cutaneous involvement; ocular lesions are especially problematic because they have a high risk of sequelae. Initially, the conjunctivae are erythematous and painful. The lids are often stuck together, with efforts to loosen them resulting in tearing of the epidermis. Pseudomembranous conjunctival erosions may form synechiae between the eyelids and the conjunctivae. Keratitis, corneal erosions, and a sicca-like syndrome may develop. Treatment of these dreaded conditions requires withdrawal of the offending drug, supportive therapy in a burn unit and pharmacologic therapy as outlined above for erythema multiforme major.

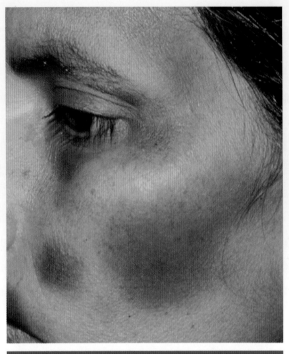

Fixed Drug Eruption

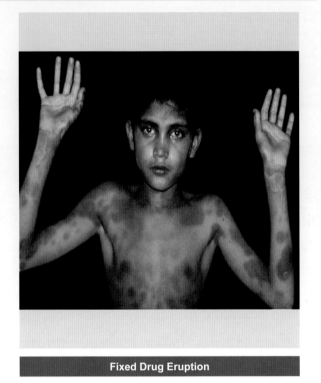

Fixed Drug Eruption

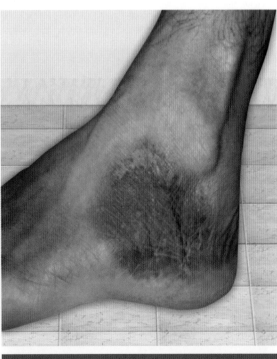

Fixed Drug Eruption

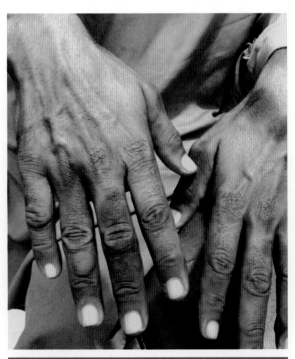

Fixed Drug Eruption

FIXED DRUG ERUPTION

The term **Fixed Drug Eruption** describes the development of one or more annular or oval erythematous patches as a result of systemic exposure to a drug; these reactions normally resolve with hyperpigmentation and may recur at the same site with re-exposure to the drug.

Several variants of fixed drug eruption have been described, based on their clinical features and the distribution of the lesions. These include the pigmenting, generalized or multiple, linear, wandering, non-pigmenting, bullous, eczematous, urticarial, erythema dyschromicum perstans-like, vulvitis, oral, psoriasiform, cellulitis-like eruption. The initial eruption is often solitary and frequently located on the lip or genitalia. Rarely, the eruption may be intraoral.

Readministration of the medication poses the risk of increased pigmentation, size, and number of lesions. Individuals with darker pigmentation may develop post-inflammatory hypopigmented macules once the lesions have resolved. Diagnosis remains clinical as blood studies are not useful for the diagnosis of fixed drug eruption (FDE), although eosinophilia is common with drug eruptions. The main goal of treatment is to identify the causative agent and avoid it. **Treatment for fixed drug eruptions** otherwise is symptomatic. Systemic antihistamines and topical corticosteroids may be all that are required. In cases in which infection is suspected, antibiotics and proper wound care are advised. Desensitization to medications has been reported in the literature, but this should be avoided unless no substitutes exist.

Chapter 4

CONNECTIVE TISSUE DISORDERS

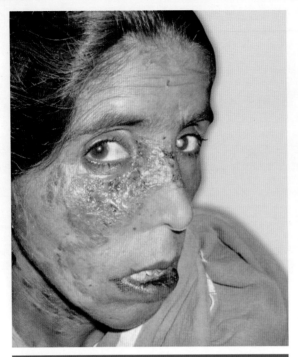

Discoid Lupus Erythematosus

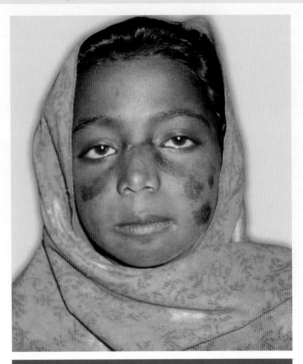

Systemic Lupus Erythematosus

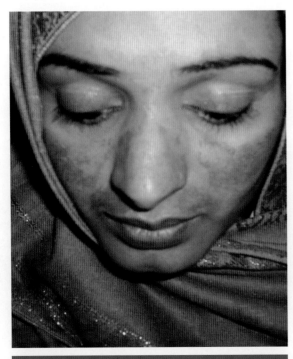

Systemic Lupus Erythematosus

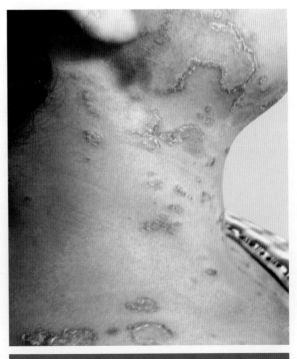

Subacute Lupus Erythematosus

SYSTEMIC LUPUS ERYTHEMATOSUS (SLE)

It is an autoimmune disorder that runs a chronic course. It can involve any organ of the body; therefore, its clinical presentations are very different, ranging from simple disease to a complicated one. In childhood SLE, the clinical symptoms such as malar rash, mucosal involvement, proteinuria/ renal involvement, urinary cellular casts, CNS involvement, low platelet count, hemolytic anemia, unexplained fever and lymphadenopathy, are usually more common as compared to the adults. In adults, Raynaud, pleuritis and sicca are twice as common as in children and adolescents. The classical symptoms of fever, joint pain, and rash (triad) in a fertile woman should lead to immediate attempts to diagnose SLE. In cases with suspicious findings, and a positive family history of autoimmune disorder should alert the physician about the presence of SLE. A conclusive diagnosis of SLE requires the presence of four out of the eleven criteria of American College of Rheumatology (ACR). The following are the ACR diagnostic criteria in SLE: Serositis, Oral ulcers, Arthritis, Photosensitivity, Blood disorders, Renal involvement, Antinuclear antibodies, Immunologic phenomena (e.g. dsDNA; anti-Smith [Sm] antibodies), Neurologic disorder, Malar rash, Discoid rash. Subacute cutaneous lupus is a rash seen in up to 10% of SLE cases, but importantly, 50% of patients with this condition will have it in isolation without systemic lupus if the characteristic appearance is an annular or *psoria* form patch with crusted margins. Lesions often occur on the limbs or torso in sun-exposed areas. Alopecia is not a specific finding of SLE. It usually occurs on the temporal regions or a patchy hair loss is seen. Other findings in SLE include the Raynaud's phenomenon, panniculitis (lupus profundus), livedo reticularis, vasculitic purpura, bullous lesions, telangiectasias and urticaria. Medications used to treat SLE include the following: Biologic DMARDs (disease-modifying antirheumatic drugs): Belimumab, rituximab, IV immunoglobulin; Nonbiologic DMARDs: Cyclophosphamide, methotrexate, azathioprine, mycophenolate, cyclosporine; NSAIDS, e.g. ibuprofen, naproxen, diclofenac; Steroids (e.g. methylprednisolone, prednisone); Antimalarials (e.g. hydroxychloroquine).

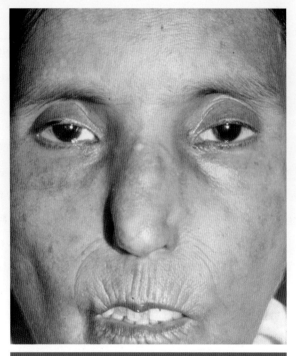

Systemic Sclerosis

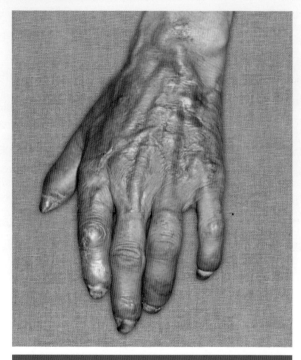

Systemic Sclerosis

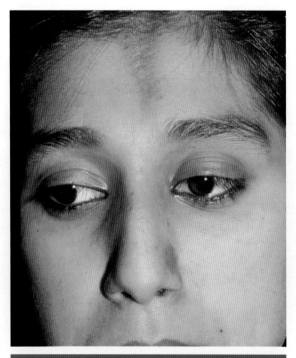

Encoup De Sabre

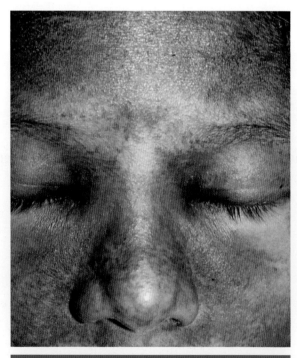

Dermatomyositis

SYSTEMIC SCLEROSIS

Systemic sclerosis is a chronic, autoimmune systemic connective tissue disease. Characteristic features are vascular abnormalities, fibrosis, subsequent atrophy of the skin, subcutaneous tissue, muscles, and internal organs such as gastrointestinal tract, lungs, heart, kidney, CNS; and immunologic abnormalities. The American College of Rheumatology (ACR) has divided the manifestations into 2 groups: Major and minor criteria. Systemic sclerosis is diagnosed when a patient has 1 major and 2 minor criteria. Major criteria is centrally located skin sclerosis that affects the arms, face, and/or neck. Minor criteria may be sclerodactyly, erosions, atrophy of the tips of digits, and bilateral fibrosis of the lungs. Cutaneous features evolve through three stages: edematous, indurative and atrophic. There are numerous telangiectasias, especially in the atrophic stage. Radial furrowing around the mouth is another characteristic finding in the later phase of the disease.

LINEAR MORPHEA

Linear morphea is characterized by thick linear bands, usually single and unilateral in most of the cases. *Frontoparietal linear morphea, known as en coup de sabre,* is typified by a linear, atrophic groove over the frontoparietal region of the scalp. Paramedian distribution of these lesions is common. They may extend into the underlying organs, leading to ocular and central nervous system symptoms. Scalp involvement results in scarring alopecia. Lesions of superficial morphea often heal spontaneously over 3–5 years. Limited disease can often be managed with topical therapy or limited phototherapy. Active lesions can be treated with potent topical or intralesional steroids. 0.1% Tacrolimus ointment, applied two times daily for 3 months may be beneficial. Topical calcipotriene may also be beneficial.

DERMATOMYOSITIS

Dermatomyositis is an autoimmune, chronic inflammatory disease mainly affecting the muscles, with specific skin features, occurring both in children and adults. Other organs that may also be affected include the esophagus, lungs, joints, and less commonly, the heart. Cutaneous features may include: an erythematous eruption on the exposed areas; Pruritus, sometimes very severe; Scaly dermatitis on the scalp or diffuse hair loss. Muscle involvement may be seen simultaneously, it may precede the cutaneous manifestations, or may follow these features by weeks, sometimes years. Muscle disease manifests as: Proximal muscle weakness. Muscle weakness while walking, going upstairs, rising from a sitting posture, combing hair, or moving the arms above shoulders. Sometimes muscle tenderness. Other systemic features that may be seen are: Arthralgia, Arthritis; Dyspnea; Dysphagia; Dysphonia; Arrhythmia and Malignancy, particularly in older patients.

Chapter 5

ICHTHYOSES

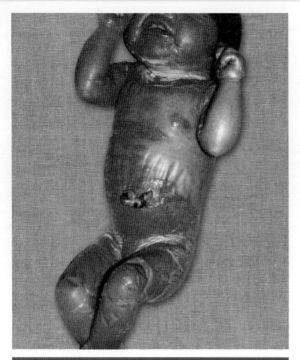

Collodion Baby

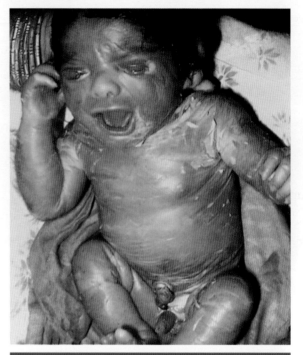

Collodion Baby. Parchment Membrance Encasing the Infant, Ectropion

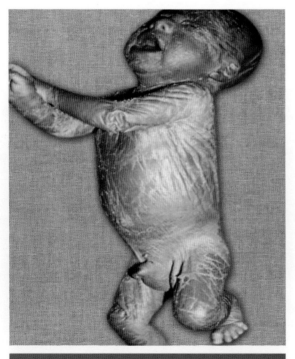

Collodion Baby

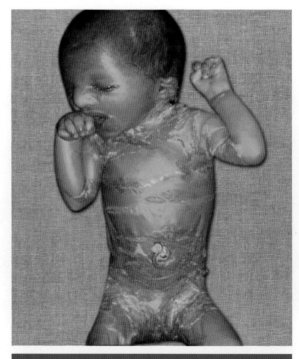

Collodion Baby

ICHTHYOSES

It is a group of relatively uncommon skin diseases, which is characterized by the clinical findings of excessive dry scaling on the skin surface. It is caused by an abnormal epidermal differentiation or metabolism and is categorized as a disorder of keratinization. The term **collodion baby** is used for newborns in whom all the body surface is covered by thick skin sheets, so called *"collodion membrane"*. It is the result of an epidermal developmental dysfunction, and is composed of thick skin sheets which resemble translucent, tight parchment paper. In almost all the cases, an autosomal recessive ichthyosiform disease is implicated. Diseases associated with collodion baby include: Autosomal recessive congenital ichthyoses [congenital ichthyosiform erythroderma (nonbullous form), lamellar ichthyosis, harlequin ichthyosis], Epidermolytic hyperkeratosis (bullous congenital ichthyosiform erythroderma). The collodion membrane limits both the baby's respiration and sucking function. The collodion membrane peels off in two or more weeks frequently leaving behind fissures and skin barrier dysfunctions. As a result, serious complications like risk of infection, fluid loss, hypernatremic dehydration, electrolyte imbalance and thermal instability may be encountered. The collodion babies are usually premature at birth. The eyelids and lips may be everted and tethered (ectropion and eclabion).

In collodion babies, fluid and electrolyte balance and body temperature must be carefully monitored. In addition to this, the membrane must be lubricated to achieve elasticity and desquamation, adequate hydration of skin is the major component of management. Suitable eye care and pain control should be carried out for the babies with ectropion. Humidified incubators and water dressings followed by emollient agents are the essentials of management. If there is a respiratory failure, ventilator support may surely be needed. In cases of epidermolytic hyperkeratosis (bullous congenital ichthyosiform erythroderma), which show generalized erythema, bullae and erosions, an antibacterial will be needed. The collodion babies with large areas of skin erosions are always under the risk of heavy infections and even sepsis, therefore suitable local and systemic antibacterial agents must be cautiously determined and preferred.

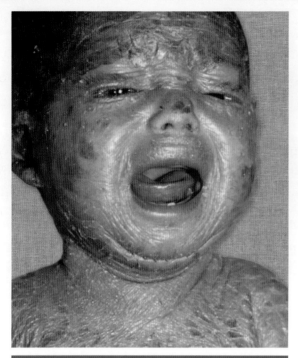

Non-bullous Ichthyosiform Erythroderma

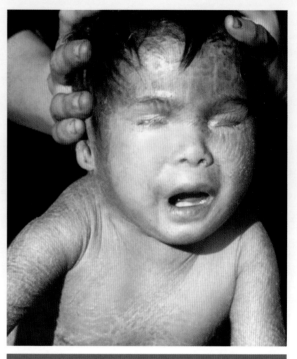

Non-bullous Ichthyosiform Erythroderma

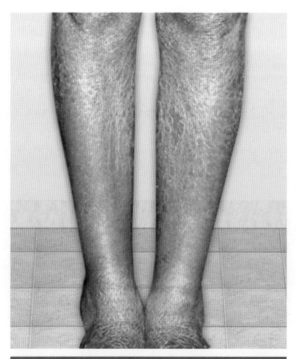

Non-bullous Ichthyosiform Erythroderma

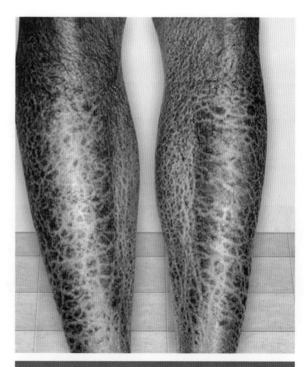

X-linked Ichthyosis

NONBULLOUS ICHTHYOSIFORM ERYTHRODERMA

Nonbullous ichthyosiform erythroderma (NBIE) or congenital ichthyosiform erythroderma (CIE) is inherited as an autosomal recessive disorder. The patients present with generalized erythema with white, thin scaling. Other features of the disease are persistent ectropion and scarring alopecia. There may be a collodion membrane encasing the neonate. As it sheds, there is underlying erythroderma (involvement of >90% of the body with an inflammatory process). It is covered with fine white scales. As the baby grows older, the erythroderma may settle and in due course, there is improvement in scaling too.

X-LINKED RECESSIVE ICHTHYOSIS

X-linked recessive ichthyosis is a type of ichthyosis, due to a mutation in the enzyme steroid sulfatase (STS). STS is involved in the metabolism of cholesterol sulfate, needed for the development of a healthy stratum corneum. Clinically, patients develop hyperkeratosis along with skin barrier dysfunction. A dirty facial appearance is produced by a widespread adherent brown scaling. Scaling on the scalp, retro-auricular area, and back of neck may manifest in early childhood. Palms and soles are usually spared, but involvement of flexures may be evident.

As regards the treatment of ichthyosis, certain keratolytic agents like salicylic acid, lactic acid and propylene glycol can be used in order to remove the hyperkeratotic sheets from the skin. But in such cases with generalized lesions, particularly in newborns, it must not be forgotten that the application of salicylic acid locally in extreme doses may cause salicylic acid toxemia. Therefore, local remedy in these cases should be cautiously monitored. However, in the collodion babies with localized lesions, local retinoic acid and calcipotriol treatments have been reported to be successful. Systemic retinoids are currently a preferred treatment method, giving impressive results in cases with generalized lesions. In cases of lamellar ichthyosis, systemic retinoids have been begun at doses of 0.5 mg/kg/day and later on the doses have eventually been increased to 2 mg/kg/day. Systemic retinoids have also shown to be effective for cases with congenital ichthyosiform erythroderma.

Chapter 6

KERATINIZATION DISORDERS

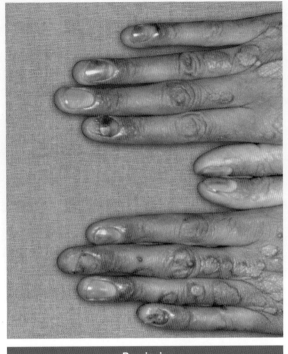

Psoriasis

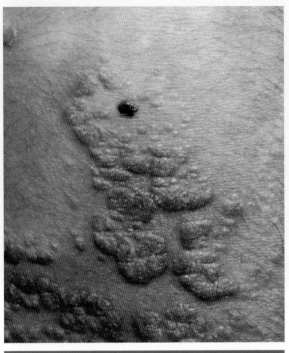

Psoriasis

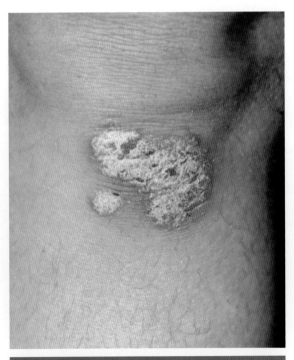

Psoriasis

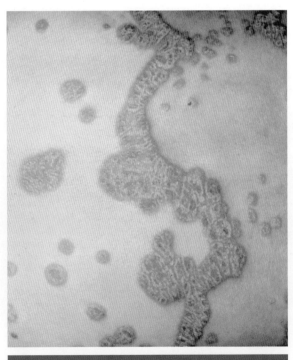

Psoriasis

PSORIASIS

Psoriasis is a common, genetically determined skin disease, often chronic, characterized by dull red lesions covered by silvery scales and not too infrequently associated with arthritis. It is probably a reaction pattern to various stimuli in a genetically predisposed person. Provocative factors include streptococcal tonsillitis (causing guttate psoriasis), other infections, stress, vaccination, sunlight, adolescence, climacteric condition and drugs, e.g. chloroquine and quinine. It can occur at any age, but is rarely seen before three years of age. Histologically, there is tortuosity of papillary capillaries, formation of intraepidermal abscesses, elongation of papillae and rete-pegs, reduction in granular layer, parakeratosis and hyperkeratosis. Typical lesions are well-defined, dull-red papules covered with silvery scales. On mild scratching, bleeding points are seen due to movement of the papillary capillaries close to the skin surface (Auspitz's sign). Classically, lesions affect extensor surfaces, e.g. elbows, knees and sacral region. Scalp may be involved alone. Palms and soles show hyperkeratosis, scaling and fissuring. Mucosal lesions are rarely present. Nail changes are common including pitting, ridging, thickening, discoloration, subungual hyperkeratosis, splinter hemorrhages, onycholysis and complete loss of nails.

In cases of psoriatic arthritis, any joint can be involved but peripheral mono- or asymmetrical oligoarthritis is the commonest. Other forms include distal interphalangeal arthritis, rheumatoid-like arthritis, arthritis mutilans, spondylitis/sacroiliitis and POPP (psoriatic onycho pachydermo periostitis). X-ray changes show osteal erosions and in severe cases gross deformities. Rheumatoid factor is absent. In Koebner's phenomenon, appearance of lesions at the site of trauma, operation scars, sunburn, vaccination or pre-existing disease is seen. It occurs in eruptive phase and is an indication for caution in therapy. There are many morphological types: Guttate (Rain drop-like), seen in children and adolescents, particularly in girls, after a sore throat. Nummular (Commonest type), rounded, disc-shaped lesions.

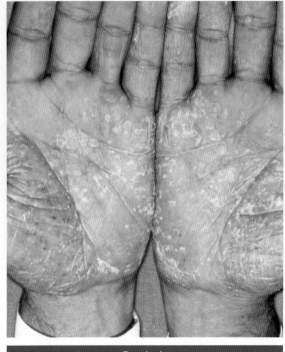

Psoriasis

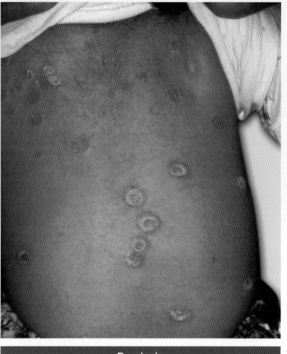

Psoriasis

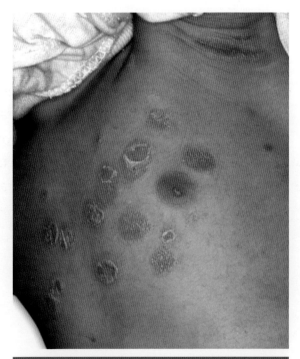

Psoriasis

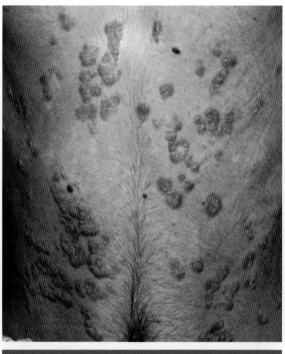

Psoriasis

Psoriasis may present as annular plaques or may take various forms during the treatment phase. Annular lesions are frequently seen, as are arciform (open circles or arcs) and, through their confluence, figurate configurations are frequently present. Annular urticarias, granuloma annulare, tinea, leprosy and secondary syphilis are important differential diagnoses at this stage. A single digit may be involved. Hands and feet can get involved due to trauma from daily shearing stresses and minor trauma resulting in isomorphic phenomenon. It is one of the causes of erythroderma, involving >90% of the body. The barrier function of skin is jeopardized resulting in increased transepidermal loss of water, electrolytes, nutrients, and heat. Similarly, there is increased peripheral circulation of blood with the resultant risk of high output cardiac failure. There may be constitutional symptoms & generalized lymphadenopathy. Histopathological findings at this stage may be non-specific.

Circinate (Ringed lesions), with clear centers and scaly margins. Rupioid (Limpet-like lesions), with cone-shaped hyperkeratosis particularly on feet. Flexural, also called psoriasis inversus because flexures are affected instead of extensor surfaces, usually seen in obese, middle-aged women. Pustular, is characterized by pustule formation in a patient with pre-existing ordinary psoriasis or arising de novo. Lesions are localized (usually to palms and soles), exanthematous or generalized. Indiscriminate use of steroids, cytotoxic drugs or sunlight may precipitate ordinary psoriasis into pustular psoriasis. Exfoliative (erythrodermic), involvement of more than 90% of skin with psoriasis due to precipitation by infections, hypocalcemia, sunlight and drugs, e.g. chloroquine. Course is stormy and chronic with considerable mortality.

ONYCHOGRYPHOSIS

Onychogryphosis, also known as **'ram's horn nails' or 'claw nails'**. There is excessive elongation, thickening, discoloration, excessive ridging, curvature and even twisting of nail plate. Poor peripheral circulation, diabetes mellitus, psoriasis, fungal infections and ichthyosis hystrix are some of its well known causes. Apart from these, ill-fitting shoes and local trauma from any cause, e.g. as seen in footballers can result in onychogryphosis. Treatment involves complete nail avulsion and carbolic or surgical destruction of the nail matrix. Cosmetic camouflage using nail polish application on the exposed nail bed can somewhat ameliorate the psychological issues resulting from nail destruction.

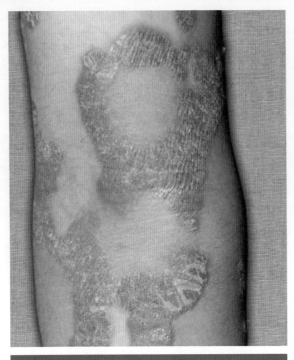

Psoriasis

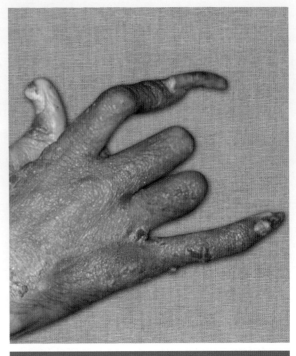

Psoriasis with Onychogryphosis

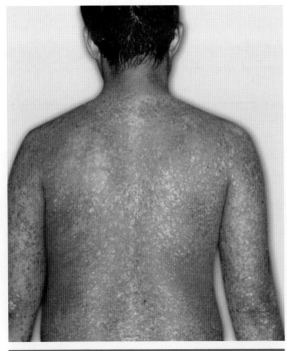

Psoriasis

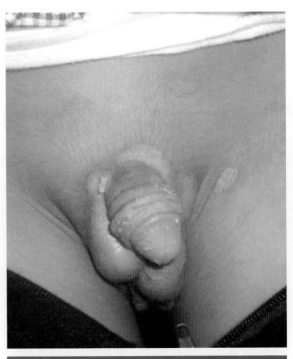

Psoriasis

Treatment

a. *General:* Proper understanding of the patient's psyche is imperative. Removal of aggravating factors is important, e.g. infection. Rest is required in all forms of unstable, pustular or exfoliative psoriasis. Tranquilizers and sedatives can be used to remove anxiety.

b. *Local:* It is the mainstay of therapy in majority of cases. In acute psoriasis, only bland preparations are used to avoid exacerbations, e.g. soft yellow paraffin, salicylated ointment or weak steroids. For chronic cases, coal and pine tars, dithranol, psoralens, calcipotriol, tazarotene or steroids with or without occlusion. Ultraviolet light is a useful adjunct.

c. *Systemic:* Cytotoxic drugs, e.g. methotrexate 10–25 mg intravenous once a week or fortnight, can also be given orally in appropriate dosage. Psoralens as part of PUVA therapy; Retinoids (Vitamin A analogues), e.g. acitretin 1 mg/kg body weight, are useful for severe forms. Combined with tar, dithranol or PUVA the dose can be lowered, hence the reduced toxicity. Cyclosporin, for severe psoriasis unresponsive to conventional therapy in a dose of 2.5 to 5 mg/ kg divided in 2 doses daily. Corticosteroids, e.g. prednisolone 5–15 mg qid initially and then gradually reduced. These can be given in erythroderma with metabolic complications, pustular psoriasis of pregnancy and mutilating arthritis.

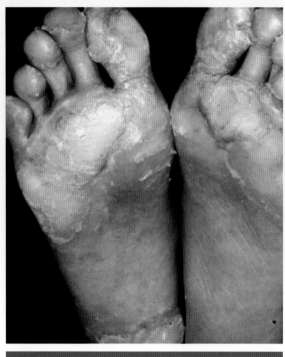

Psoriasis

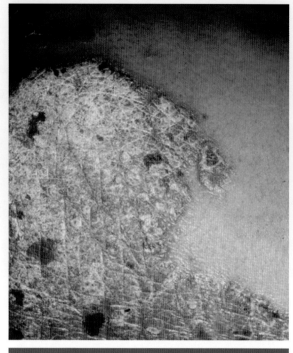

Psoriasis

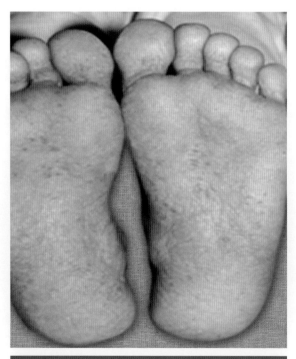

Punctate Keratoderma

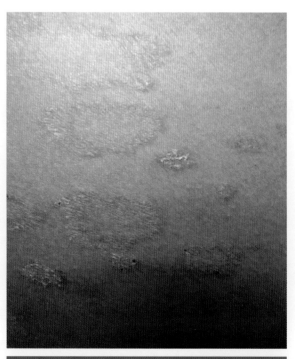

Pityriasis Rosea

PUNCTATE KERATODERMA

There are many causes of Punctate Keratoderma, e.g. Psoriasis, Pityriasis Rubra Pilaris, Warts, Porokeratosis of Mibelli, Darier's disease and Arsenical keratosis, etc. It may be due to genetically determined autosomal dominant condition.

PITYRIASIS ROSEA

It is an acute, self-limiting, idiopathic skin disease, characterized by typical skin eruption and insignificant systemic symptoms. Exact etiology is unknown but on epidemiological and clinical grounds, viral etiology is possible. Both sexes are susceptible between the ages of 10 and 35. Initial lesion is a sharply demarcated, round or oval, erythematous scaly plaque, larger than any subsequent lesion (called herald patch since it heralds the onset of eruption) 2–5 cm in diameter. It is usually found on thighs, upper arms, trunk or neck. General eruption follows in 5–15 days, occurring in crops. Classically, discrete, dull pink, oval plaques are seen with clear centers and a marginal collarette of fine, dry, gray scales. Long axis of lesions are typically parallel to the ribs. Occasionally eruption is entirely macular. Mucosal involvement is rare. Itching is mild to moderate. Constitutional symptoms may be absent. Occasionally there is mild pyrexia, malaise or lymphadenopathy. Skin lesions, as a rule appear in 3–6 weeks but may take longer. Differential diagnosis includes seborrheic dermatitis, drug eruption, secondary syphilis and guttate psoriasis. Topical steroids can be used and ultraviolet light for resistant cases.

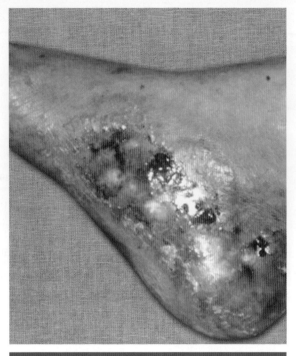

Lichen Planus

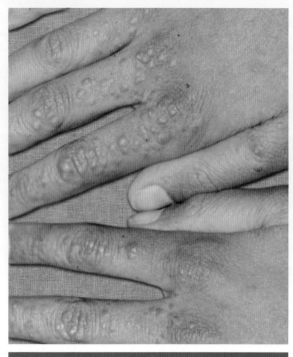

Lichen Planus

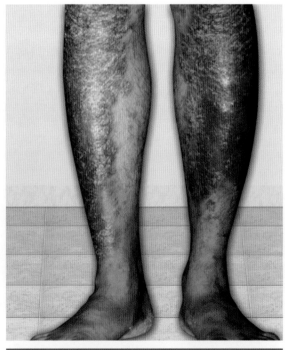

Lichen Planus

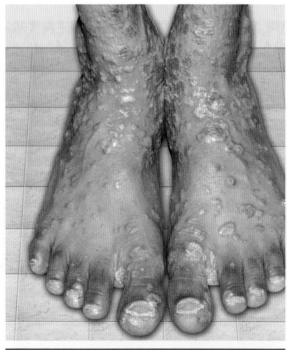

Lichen Planus

LICHEN PLANUS

It is an idiopathic mucocutaneous disorder characterized by pruritic, plane-topped, purplish, polygonal, papules and plaques. The latter are sometimes called the 5 or 6 'Ps' of lichen planus. Its sites of predilection include the oral mucosa, tongue, wrists, nails, ankles and may also involve the scalp resulting in scarring alopecia. It is associated with hepatitis C virus infection, liver disease from any other cause, renal failure, diabetes mellitus, graft versus host disease and certain drugs. However, a causal relationship with any of these remains elusive. The purplish color of the papules results from a deeper, dermal deposition of pigment. The whitish reticular pattern on the surface owes its appearance to a patchy thickening of stratum granulosum. Its gross appearance is called Wickham's striae. When lichen planus affects the buccal, gingival or the vaginal mucosa, these striae are thought to be the sites of origin of squamous cell carcinoma. Though totally different from psoriasis, lichen planus also demonstrates the Koebner's or reverse Koebner's phenomenon. Ankles and dorsa of feet show numerous papules and plaques typical of lichen planus. Upon histopathology, there is compact hyperkeratosis, patchy hypergranulosis, presence of colloid bodies in the spinous layer, basal cell degeneration with pigmentary incontinence and a saw-tooth appearance of the rete pegs. The papillary dermis shows a band-like lymphocytic infiltrate. When inflammation is intense, the dermoepidermal junction may show separation and vesiculation, these spaces are called Max Joseph spaces.

In acute case, bed rest, antihistamines, sedatives and local steroids are used. In ordinary lichen planus, oral antihistamines and local steroids are useful. In hypertrophic lichen planus, local steroids under occlusion, intralesional steroids and oral antihistamines can be used. Mucosal lesions require topical triamcinolone in orabase and watch over the years for malignancy. Treatments aimed at immunomodulation include topical UVB, systemic steroids, antimalarials, dapsone, retinoids, azathioprine, etc. Disease course is prolonged and healing leaves behind post-inflammatory hyperpigmentation that lasts a long time.

Chapter 7

GENODERMATOSES

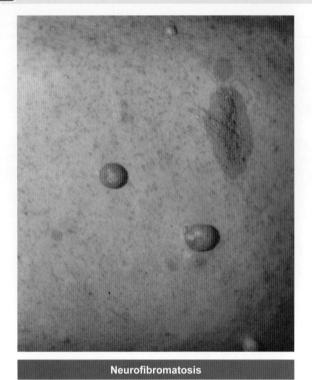

Neurofibromatosis

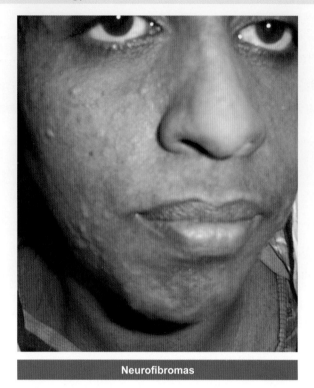

Neurofibromas

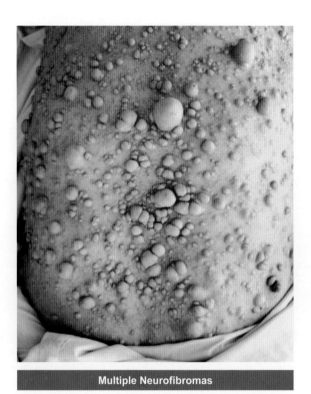

Multiple Neurofibromas

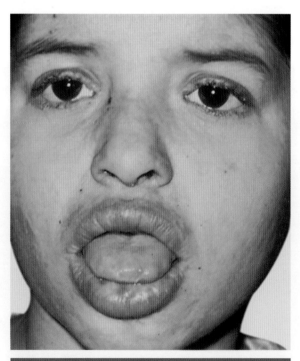

Lipoid Proteinosis: Moniliform Blepharosis, Yellowish White Plaques Oral Cavity, Face

NEUROFIBROMATOSIS

Neurofibromatosis also called von Recklinghausen's disease, is a neuroectodermal disorder inherited as autosomal dominant trait. Light brown cafe au lait spots, often more than five, are characteristically present. Pigmented macules on axillary apices and perineum, found in one-fifth of cases, are considered more pathognomonic. Soft, lilac-pink, sessile and sometimes pedunculated tumors appear along the peripheral nerves. Their size and number varies. Skin tumors are often asymptomatic but intracranial tumors like optic nerve gliomas and acoustic neuromas may cause pressure symptoms. NF1 is diagnosed on the basis of the presence of two of the key points: Presence of at least 6 Cafe au lait spots, ≥ 2 neurofibromas of any type or 1 plexiform neurofibroma, freckling in the axillae and groins, first degree relative with NF1, optic glioma, Lisch nodules (2 or more) and definite bone lesions. Treatment is symptomatic. Surgery is required for disfiguring lesions or when sarcomatous change is suspected.

LIPOID PROTEINOSIS

Lipoid proteinosis usually presents in infancy with hoarseness. There are yellow, waxy infiltrations of the face, eyelids, elsewhere on skin and lips, secondary to deposits of an amorphous hyaline material. Oral cavity, larynx and internal organs are also involved. At present, there is no curative therapy for this disorder, although some of its symptoms can be managed. Oral dimethyl sulfoxide (DMSO), D-penicillamine, etretinate and intralesional heparin have shown some benefit in few cases. Laser therapy with CO_2 Laser for thickened vocal cords and beaded eyelid papules has shown some promise. As it has been discovered that there are mutations in the ECM1 gene, it has led to the possibility of gene therapy or a recombinant EMC1 protein for this disorder.

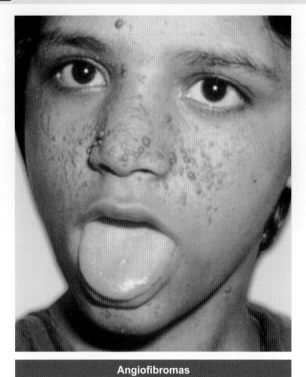

Angiofibromas

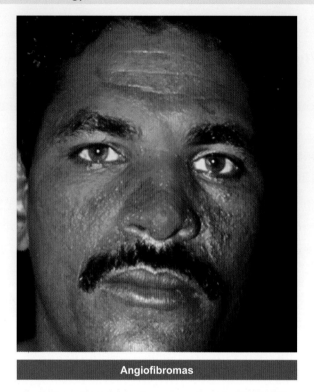

Angiofibromas

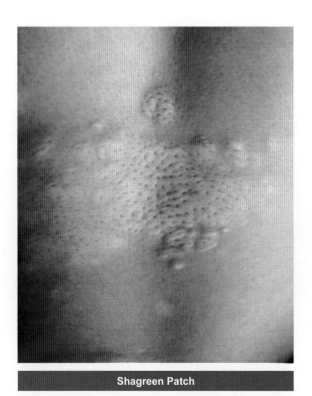

Shagreen Patch

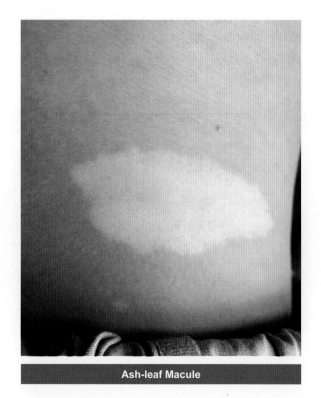

Ash-leaf Macule

TUBEROUS SCLEROSIS

Tuberous sclerosis also known as **Epiloia, Adenoma sebaceum, Pringle's disease** and **Bournville's disease**. There is a widespread connective tissue defect which shows an autosomal dominant inheritance with variable penetration. The onset occurs before the age of five usually with skin changes or epilepsy. Cutaneous lesions include adenoma sebaceum which are discrete, firm, pink, telangiectatic papules on nose, cheeks and chin. Shagreen patches are soft, irregularly thickened plaques usually seen in lumbosacral region. Koenen's tumors are firm, skin-colored and periungual fibromata. White macules are ovoid or Ash leaf-shaped lesions, best seen under Wood's light. Neurological features include epilepsy and mental deficiency. Other systems may also be affected. In the absence of any curative treatment, only symptomatic measures are available.

More than five ash leaf macules in an infant are highly suggestive. Confetti spots are virtually pathognomonic. Family members of the patient should be thoroughly studied and imaging studies of various types as well as electroencephalography should be obtained. There may not be any mental retardation or seizures. The associations are CNS (tumors producing seizures), eye (gray or yellow retinal plaques, 50%) heart (benign rhabdomyomas), hamartomas of mixed cell type (kidney, liver, thyroid, testes, and GI system). The management includes prevention by counseling and treatment of angiofibromas by electrofulguration and laser surgery.

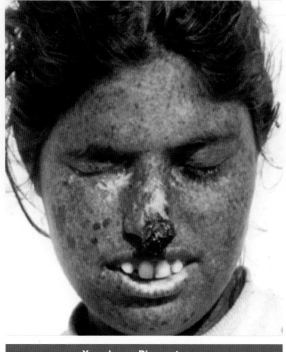

Xeroderma Pigmentosum

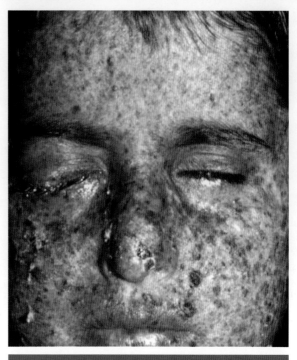

Xeroderma Pigmentosum

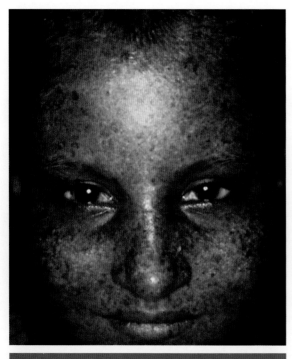

Xeroderma Pigmentosum

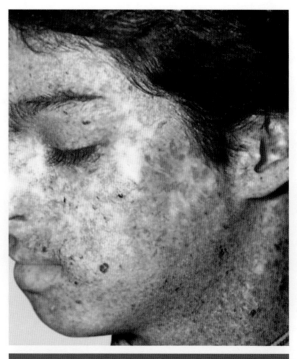

Xeroderma Pigmentosum

XERODERMA PIGMENTOSUM

Xeroderma pigmentosum is an autosomal recessive disorder, which is characterized by dryness, pigmentation, keratotic and neoplastic changes in the skin mainly on the exposed areas. It is caused by defective repair of the damage to DNA by ultraviolet light. Symptoms first appear six months after birth but sometimes later. Freckling and dryness on sun exposed sites are seen followed by telangiectasis and white atrophic macules. Indolent ulcers result in scarring. Malignant changes may appear in early childhood or later, in the form of BCC, SCC or melanoma. Death may occur in majority of cases before the age of twenty.

Treatment

Photoprotection is most improtant, strictly avoid sunlight. Use protective clothing. Regular use of sunscreens round the clock. Tumor surveillance and removal of overt neoplasia is essential. Topical retinoic acid and systemic retinoids are useful in the prevention of neoplasia.

Chapter 8

ECZEMAS

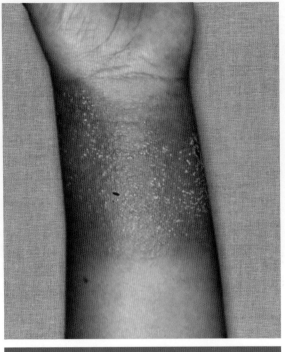

Allergic Contact Dermatitis

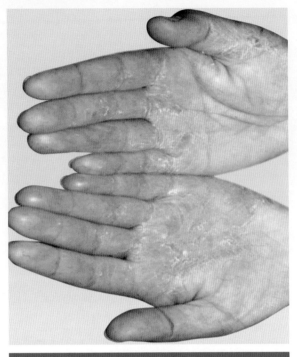

Contact Dermatitis

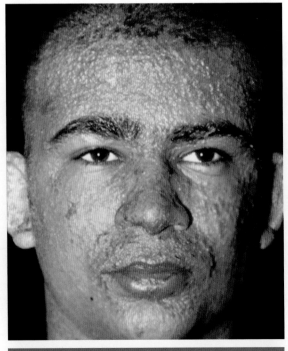

Contact Dermatitis

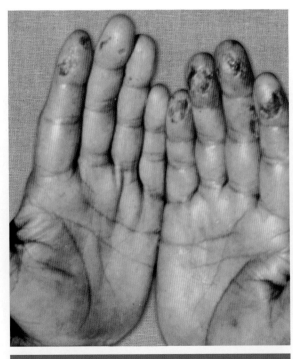

Contact Dermatitis

ECZEMA

Eczema is a distinctive reaction of the epidermis to various agents, both endogenous and exogenous, characterized clinically by eruption of itchy, erythematous papules and vesicles leading to weeping and/or lichenification, and histological evidence of spongiosis. The terms "Dermatitis" and "Eczema" are mostly used synonymously. Dermatitis simply means inflammation of skin and is vague being used as prefix or postfix in many skin diseases, e.g. dermatitis herpetiformis, dermatitis artefacta, napkin dermatitis, etc. Eczema means "to boil" and aptly describes the condition in which vesicles are thrown up by epidermis just like bubbles rising after boiling. Every eczema is a dermatitis, but every dermatitis is not eczema.

CONTACT DERMATITIS

Contact dermatitis is the type of eczema due to contact with external agents. It is divided into *Irritant Contact Dermatitis (ICD)* and *Allergic Contact Dermatitis (ACD)*. An irritant is a substance which can produce damage if applied in adequate concentrations for a sufficient period of time. ICD occurs if the body cannot repair this cell damage. Strong irritants elicit an acute response usually after one application, e.g. sulphuric acid. Weak irritants, e.g. cement and soap, produce reaction on repeated exposures called *Cumulative Insult Dermatitis*. ICD is strictly limited to the area of contact. Any part of the skin can be affected but hands and forearms are mostly involved. Allergic contact dermatitis occurs in only those who have an allergy to a contactant, e.g. nickel, hair dye, rubber, etc.

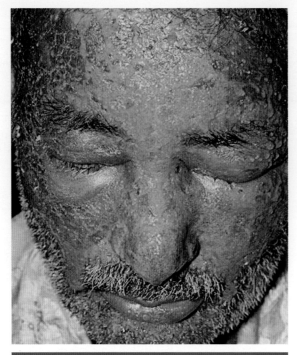

Contact Dermatitis (Chemical)

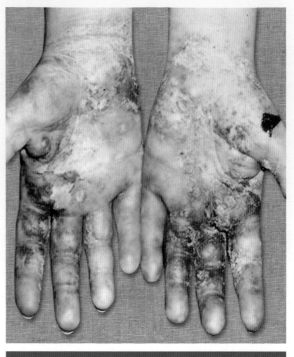

Contact Dermatitis (Chemical)

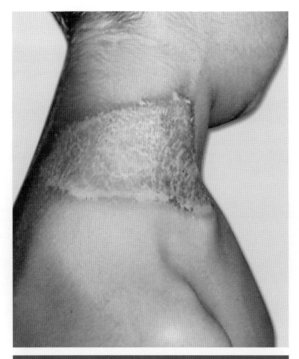

Contact Dermatitis, Dischromia Lichenification

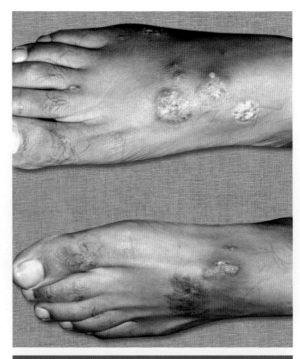

Contact Dermatitis (Shoe)

Most allergens are simple chemicals and act as haptens. Allergic contact dermatitis (ACD) is mediated by lymphocytes (delayed hypersensitivity) and is not dose related. Clinical features depend upon factors like type of allergen, site, intensity of exposure and level of sensitivity. Initial signs are erythema, edema, papule or vesicle formation and weeping. Eczema may spread away from the original site. Itching is often pronounced. Chronic cases show dryness, scaling, lichenification and fissuring. The eruption starts in a sensitized individual 48 hours or 2 days after contact with the allergen. The site of the eruption is confined to size of exposure. There is intense pruritus, in severe reaction.

Contact allergens are diverse and range from metal salts to antibiotics, dyes to plant products. Thus, allergens are found in jewelry, personal care products, topical medications, plants, house remedies, and chemicals with which the individual may come in contact at work. The most common sensitizers are Nickel, Neomycin, Bacitracin, Balsam of Peru, Sodium Gold Thiosulfate, Thimerosal, Quaternium-15 and Formaldehyde, etc. Patch testing with suspected allergen is an important diagnostic procedure.

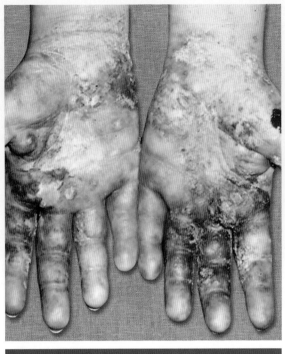

Contact Dermatitis

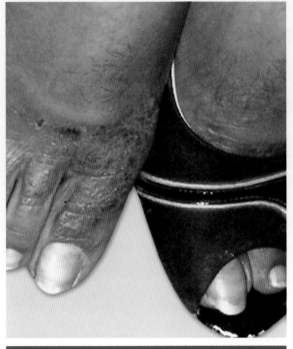

Contact Dermatitis

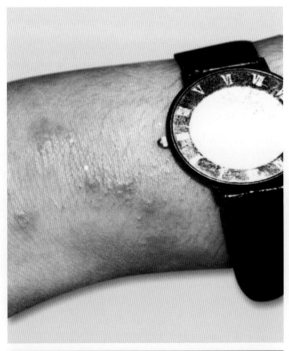

Contact Dermatitis

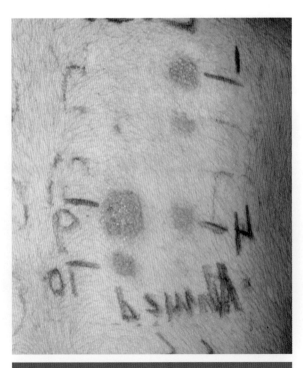

Patch Test

PATCH TEST

Patch test is the scientific procedure which is used to find out the causative substance of an allergic contact dermatitis. Patch testing is performed in an individual who is suspected of suffering from allergic contact dermatitis. It produces a local allergic reaction on a limited area of the body usually the back of patient where the suspected chemicals are applied in specific concentrations. The allergens included in the patch test series are the culprits in approximately 90% of allergic contact dermatitis and comprise of chemicals in leather, hair dyes, metals, e.g. nickel and cobalt, rubber, lanolin, fragrance, formaldehyde, preservatives and other additives.

Treatment

Treatment of both ICD and ACD includes removing the patient away from the injurious substance in question. Avoid irritants by wearing protective clothing (i.e. goggles, shields and gloves). If contact to a chemical takes place, the area should be washed with water or a weak neutralizing solution and then the barrier creams can be applied. In occupational ICD that persists, change of job may be necessary. Symptomatic treatment includes antihistamines and topical steroids and is same as for any other form of eczema.

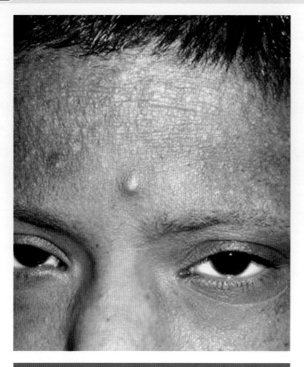

Atopic Dermatitis

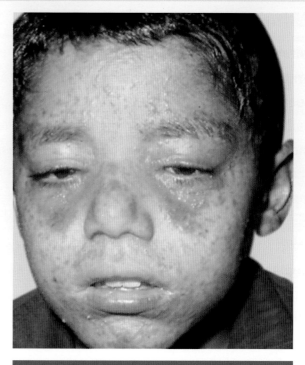

Atopic Dermatitis

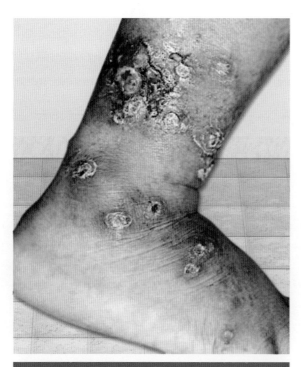

Infective Eczema

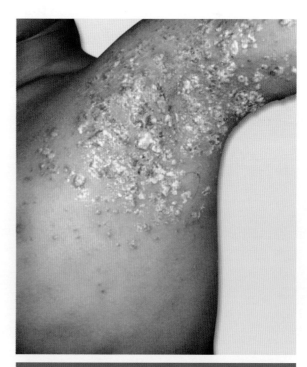

Infective Eczema

ATOPIC DERMATITIS

"**Atopy**" implies genetically determined disorders with increased liability to form reagins (IgE antibodies) and enhanced susceptibility to certain diseases like asthma, hay fever and atopic dermatitis in which such antibodies may play some role. A person suffering from this condition has an inherently itchy skin resulting in majority of the clinical features, perhaps modified by psychological, climatic and allergic factors. There is family history of atopy in 70% of cases. White dermographism (blanching of skin on stroking instead of normal erythema) is prominent. It is a chronic disease, occurring at any age. It is more common in boys. Usually starts in infancy between the age of 2–6 months. In the infantile phase, face is most frequently affected. Picture usually of a chubby child with weeping and crusting of cheeks, forehead, scalp, limbs and occasionally napkin area may be seen. Secondary infection is common. Antecubital and popliteal fossae, sides of neck, wrists and ankles are the sites of predilection in older children. In general treatment, reassurance is essential. Basic principle is to forestall itching. Avoid irritants like soap, wool, etc. and also drugs known to produce anaphylaxis, e.g. penicillins and ATS. Systemically, antihistamines e.g. promethazine and cetirizine can be used. Topical steroids with or without antibiotics may be used and coal tar paste is used in chronic lichenified cases.

INFECTIVE ECZEMA

Infective eczema is a form of eczema caused by bacterial infection not attributed to the specific pathogenic activities of the microorganisms (should be differentiated from infected eczema which means simple infection of pre-existing eczema). Erythema, exudation and crusting predominantly affect flexures. Edges of lesions are well-defined, often surmounted by small pustules. People with seborrheic diathesis are more prone. Lack of hygiene, hyperhidrosis, maceration, scratching and trauma are other factors.

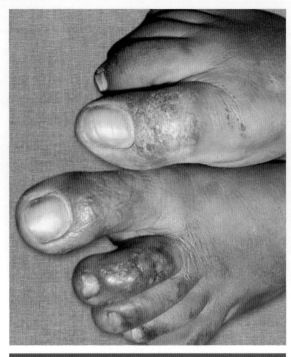

Infective Eczema

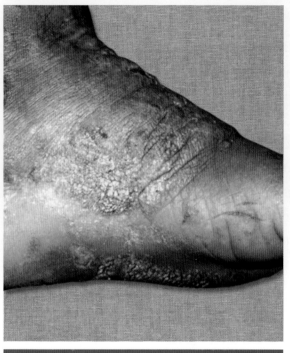

Chronic Eczema

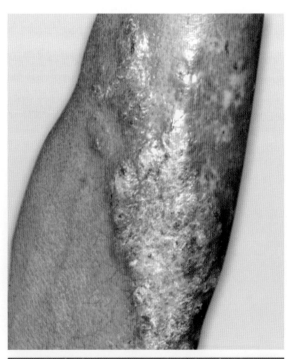

Lichen Simplex Chronicus

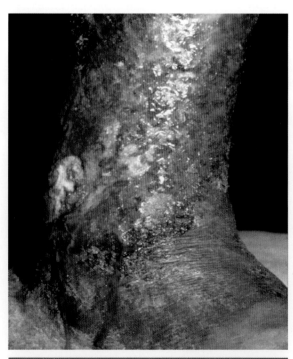

Stasis Eczema

LICHEN SIMPLEX

Lichen simplex skin usually responds to repeated rubbing by lichenification, a feature of many dermatoses e.g. atopic dermatitis, varicose eczema, etc. Lichenification arising on previously normal skin, is called lichen simplex. Emotional tension is an important etiological factor. Paroxysmal itching is a hallmark. Initially skin is red and edematous, later lichenified, scaly and pigmented. Once lichenification appears, rubbing and scratching becomes self-perpetuated. Frequently involved sites are nape of neck, lower legs, vulva, pubis, scrotum, ankles, upper thighs, scalp and extensor aspects of forearms. Differential diagnosis includes psoriasis and lichen planus hypertrophicus. Treatment is basically aimed at breaking the itch scratch reflex. Sedatives and psychotherapy are useful. Local steroids particularly under occlusion and intradermal steroid injections for circumscribed chronic lesions are useful.

STASIS ECZEMA

Stasis eczema is secondary to venous hypertension, usually in the lower leg. It develops suddenly or insidiously accompanied by edema, purpura, ulceration and atrophie blanche. Elevation of the legs should be done for a few hours daily. Mild steroids can be given for topical use. Antibiotics are sometimes needed.

Chapter 9

MISCELLANEOUS DISORDERS

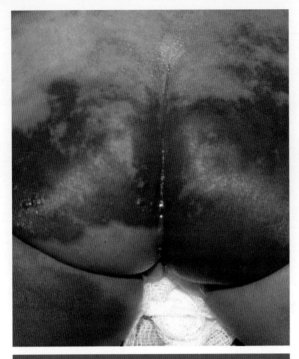

Purpura Fulminans

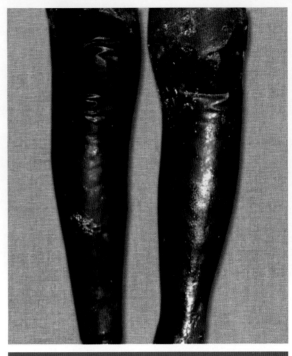

Purpura Fulminans

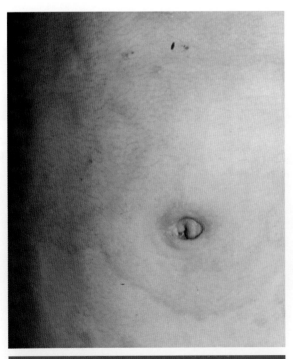

Urticaria

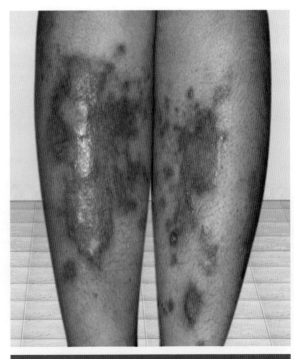

Necrobiosis Lipoidica Diabeticorum

PURPURA FULMINANS

It is a hemorrhagic condition occurring mainly in babies and small children. It is an acute emergency which manifests as skin necrosis and disseminated intravascular coagulation (DIC). Purpura fulminans can result in a rapid failure of different organ systems produced by thrombotic occlusion of blood vessels of small and medium size. Common causes are aggressive infection especially meningococcal meningitis. Some cases of severe inherited deficiency of the anticoagulants protein C or S, may also present with purpura fulminans. An early diagnosis and treatment of this condition is of utmost importance to minimize the mortality and prevent complications.

URTICARIA (HIVES)

It is characterized by the sudden appearance of pale red swellings, patches, or weals, either due to allergies or due to some other factors. Urticaria generally produces itching but can also cause burning or stinging. Any area of the body can be involved, including the face, ears, lips, tongue, or throat. Urticarial weals are of different sizes and may be closely set to form large plaques. They may last for hours, or several days before disappearing. Most common offending agents are foods, medicines, infections, insect bites, internal disease or latex. Among the foods, mostly implicated items are nuts, fish, eggs, tomatoes, chocolate, fresh berries, milk, soy, and wheat. Some food preservatives and additives may also be responsible.

NECROBIOSIS LIPOIDICA

This disorder manifests as a process of degeneration of collagen along with a granulomatous response, thickening of blood vessel walls, and deposition of fat. The disease has been renamed as *necrobiosis lipoidica diabeticorum (NLD)*. Diabetic microangiopathy may be caused by a deposition of glycoprotein in the blood vessel walls. In necrobiosis lipoidica, there is deposition of a similar glycoprotein. Skin manifestations start with small (1–3 mm), circumscribed papules that enlarge to form plaques with activity at the margin, and waxy, atrophic scarred centers. Common sites are the pretibial areas, but it can also occur on the face, trunk, scalp, and upper extremities. Telangiectatic vessels running on the surface of the lesion can be easily recognized.

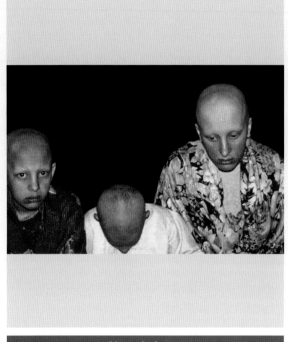

Alopecia Areata

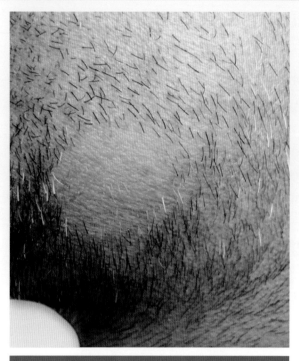

Alopecia Areata

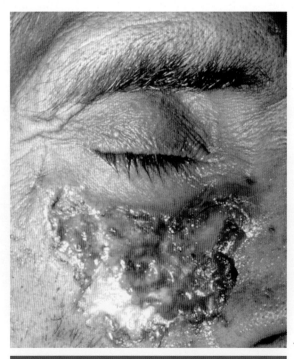

Basal Cell Carcinoma

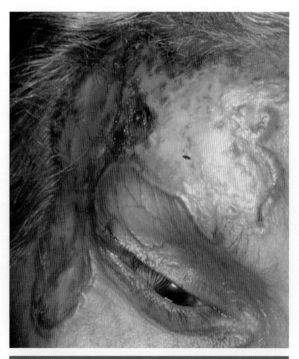

Basal Cell Carcinoma

ALOPECIA AREATA (AA)

It is an autoimmune disorder, which mostly occurs in patients of 30–60 years. The classical symptom is an area of hairless skin surrounded by areas of normal hair growth. There may be some other features that can help in making a diagnosis of AA, these are: the appearance of short hair which represent the fractured hair, yellowish areas of deposition at the follicular orifices, thin short hair, and gray hair, all seen in a bald patch. The course of typical alopecia areata is not predictable with a high likelihood of spontaneous remission. The commonest presentation is of a single or multiple patches of hair loss on the scalp. Sometimes, a diffuse thinning of hair is seen which is known as as *diffuse alopecia areata*. When hair from all over the scalp is lost, it is termed *alopecia totalis*. Rarely, loss of hair occurs on the entire body, this is called *alopecia universalis*. Intralesional corticosteroid injections, creams, lotions and shampoos have been used for a long time, over the scalp. Topical minoxidil can also be used. In some cases, oral steroids have to be given.

BASAL CELL CARCINOMA (BCC)

It is a cutaneous cancer which grows slowly. BCC is a non-melanoma skin cancer. It originates from the epidermis. Most of these carcinomas appear on the light exposed areas of skin, including the scalp. It mostly affects people of ≥ 40 years. For confirmation of diagnosis, a skin biopsy should always be taken. Management depends on the location, size and depth of the skin cancer, along with over all health of the patient. Treatment options include excision, curettage, electrodesiccation, cryotherapy, imiquimod or 5-fluorouracil for superficial BCC, Moh's microsurgery, photodynamic therapy and radiation therapy.

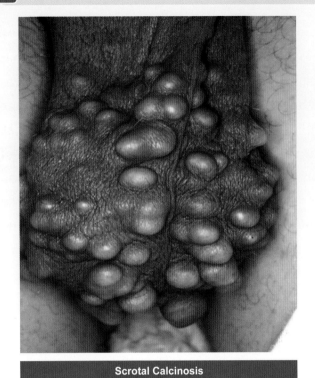

Scrotal Calcinosis

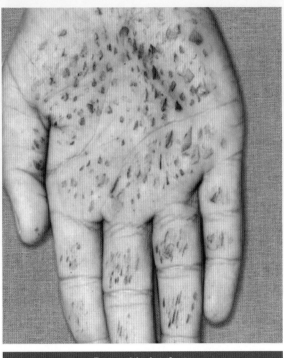

Dermatitis Artefacta

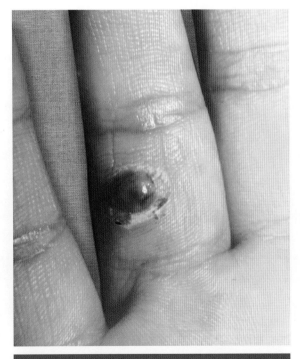

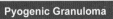
Pyogenic Granuloma

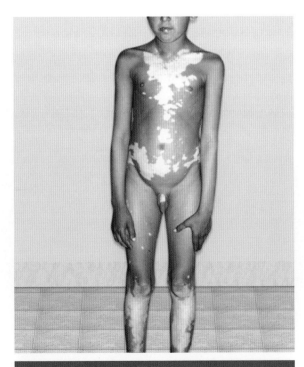

Vitiligo

CALCINOSIS

Calcinosis is characterized by deposition of calcium in the skin, subcutis, muscles and visceral organs. When the condition is localized to the skin, it is called **calcinosis cutis** or **cutaneous calcification**. Cutaneous calcification is divided into 4 types depending upon the original cause of the symptoms: **Dystrophic calcinosis cutis** occurs in the area of damaged, inflamed, necrotic or neoplastic skin. Tissue damage may have been caused by mechanical, chemical, infectious or other factors. Serum calcium and phosphate levels are within normal limits. Precipitating factors for calcinosis cutis may be trauma, infections, acne, tumors (pilomatrixoma, cysts, BCC and others), varicose veins, connective tissue disease (dermatomyositis, systemic sclerosis, SLE), panniculitis, inherited diseases of connective tissue (Ehlers-Danlos syndrome, Werner syndrome, Pseudoxanthoma elasticum, Rothmund-Thomson syndrome).

DERMATITIS ARTEFACTA (DA)

In this condition, the cutaneous lesions are self-inflicted or produced by the patients themselves. The underlying cause is psychological disturbance. A common situation may be that of an attention-seeking behavior. DA is more frequently encountered in women, mostly in their teens or early adulthood. The clinical presentation does not conform to any well known dermatosis, with bizarre-shaped lesions having an irregular outline in a linear or geometric fashion; generally easily distinguished from the surrounding normal skin.

PYOGENIC GRANULOMA

Pyogenic granuloma (PG) also known as '**granuloma telangiectaticum**', it is a common growth that presents as a shiny red mass on the skin. Its surface is raspberry-like or has a raw minced-meat appearance. Generally, it is a benign skin condition, but pyogenic granulomas may cause problems and sometimes bleed profusely. It is an idiopathic condition. The lesions of pyogenic granuloma bleed easily and may ulcerate leading to crusted lesions. Various therapeutic procedures can be employed to remove them, including curettage and cauterization, laser surgery, cryosurgery, chemical ablation using silver nitrate, and imiquimod. Recurrences are common because of the extension of feeding blood vessels into the dermis. In such cases, the most efficacious procedure would be to completely remove the affected area (excision), and close it with stitches.

VITILIGO

Vitiligo is a disorder that leads to depigmentation of areas of skin. It occurs due to the non-functioning of melanocytes, the cells which are responsible for cutaneous pigmentation. It is an idiopathic disease, but

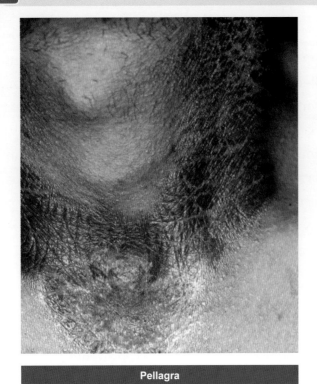

Pellagra

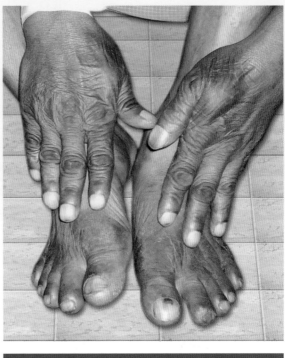

Pellagra

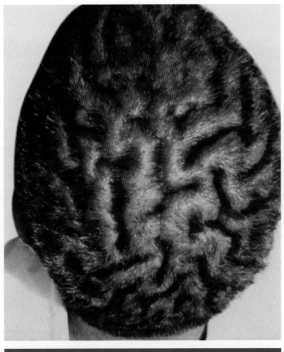

Cutis Verticis Gyrata

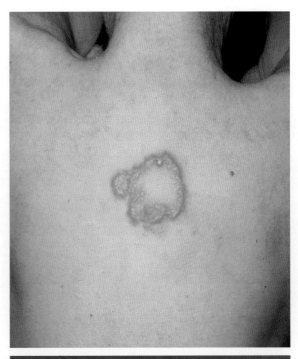

Granuloma Annulare

researchers suggests that it may be produced by genetic, autoimmune, oxidative stress, neural or viral causes. The prevalence in general population is 0.5-1%, and all races are affected. In 50% cases of vitiligo, loss of pigment starts before 20 years of age. Family history is positive in one-fifth of the patients. Both sexes are equally affected. Vitiligo of recent onset gives best results especially when it affects the face and trunk. Pigment cells surviving in the hair follicles provide pigment during healing phase, or alternatively it is derived from melanocyte stem cells. Therapies include topical steroids, calcineurin inhibitors such as topical pimecrolimus and tacrolimus, photochemotherapy and narrowband UVB phototherapy.

PELLAGRA

Pellagra is a disease characterized by diarrhea, dermatitis and dementia. It is most frequently produced by a chronic deficiency of niacin (vitamin B3) in the diet. It can arise as a result of a decreased intake of niacin or tryptophan and probably due to an excessive intake of leucine. If left untreated, the deficiency can be lethal within 4-5 years. Management is with nicotinamide, the amount and frequency of administration depends on the stage of the disease.

CUTIS VERTICIS GYRATA

Cutis verticis gyrata (CVG) is a condition characterized by multiple convoluted folds and deep furrows on the scalp which resemble the surface of brain. The condition usually runs a progressive course. A rare complication may by malignant melanoma, that develops within a melanocytic nevus. CVG mostly affects males, usually after puberty. Some of the secondary forms like cerebriform intradermal nevus, can be seen at birth. Cutis verticis gyrata classically occurs in the center and back of scalp, but some cases can involve the whole of scalp. Management strategy includes good hygiene of the scalp to avoid accumulation of secretions in the furrows. Larger lesions can be serially excised, requiring multiple surgeries.

GRANULOMA ANNULARE

Granuloma annulare (GA) is a common disorder of idiopathic origin, affecting the skin in the form of red bumps arranged in a circle or ring. GA can involve any site of the body and may be widespread in some cases. It will often disappear without leaving a scar, after a few weeks or months, but it can recur at the same site or somewhere else. Therefore, mostly no treatment is required. A strong topical steroid or an intralesional steroid injection is generally helpful. Cryotherapy can be done on small plaques or they can be removed by laser surgery. Other modes of treatment may be topical imiquimod and topical calcineurin inhibitors (tacrolimus and pimecrolimus). Some help is obtained in cases of disseminated granuloma annulare by the following agents: Systemic steroids, Methotrexate, Isotretinoin, Dapsone,

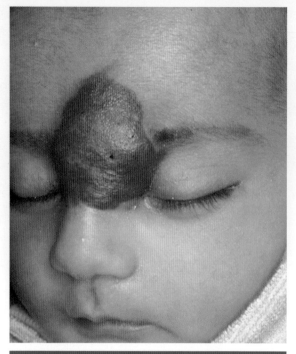

Strawberry Hemangioma

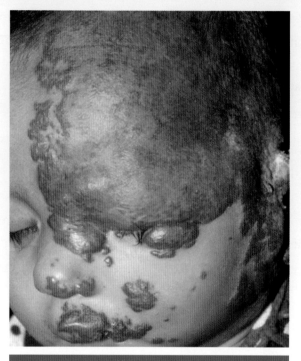

Hemangioma

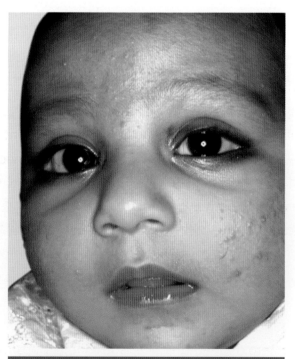

Neonatal Acne

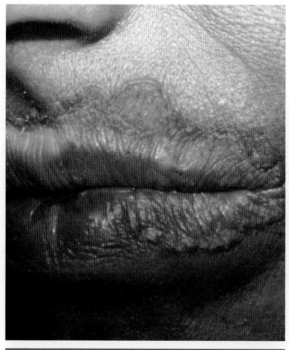

Porokeratosis of Mibelli

Potassium iodide, Hydroxychloroquine, Allopurinol, Pentoxifylline, Photochemotherapy (PUVA), and a Combination of antibiotics once monthly (rifampicin, ofloxacin, minocycline).

INFANTILE HEMANGIOMA

Infantile hemangioma is a benign disorder, affecting the blood vessels of skin. It is also called proliferative hemangioma due to the proliferation of endothelial cells. It may be seen shortly after birth. They are different from the vascular anomalies, that are less common and usually found at birth. Head and neck area is involved in > 80% of cases. They attain a maximum size in the first 3 months and most of them stop growing at about fifth month. Sometimes, they may keep on growing for up to 18 months. After that, they may undergo involution.

NEONATAL ACNE

Neonatal acne is an eruption in newborns or infants that mimics acne. It mostly appears on the nose and adjoining cheeks. The etiology is unknown, but it may be caused by the increased sensitivity of the baby's oil glands to maternal hormones during pregnancy. Classically, the peak occurrence is around two months of age and it does not require any treatment.

POROKERATOSIS OF MIBELLI

Porokeratosis is defined by the presence of cutaneous lesions characterized by a thin center with a surrounding ridge-like border known as the ***cornoid lamella***. This border is produced by an expanding group of unusual keratinocytes. Porokeratosis of Mibelli generally affects younger children, while the lesions may be found at birth or may appear at puberty for the first time. The lesions of Porokeratosis of Mibelli appear as small, light-brown, scaly papules that may join to form plaques with irregular margins. Each of these lesions has a rim as mentioned above with well-defined thin furrows in its center. Porokeratosis of Mibelli mostly occurs on the limbs especially the hands and feet, shoulders and neck, face and genitals. It may involve any part of the body including the mucous membranes. The plaques can remain silent for many years or may slowly grow to attain a larger size. A carcinoma can occur within the lesions. Treatment consists of 5-Fluorouracil cream, Calcipotriol cream, oral Acitretin or Isotretinoin, Cryotherapy, Dermabrasion, Carbon dioxide laser ablation.

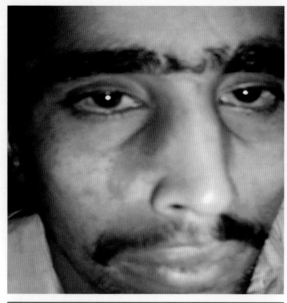

Port-Wine Stain

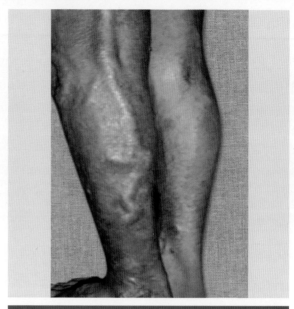

**Klippel-Trenaunay Syndrome: Portwine Stain,
Varicosities, Limb Hyperttrophy**

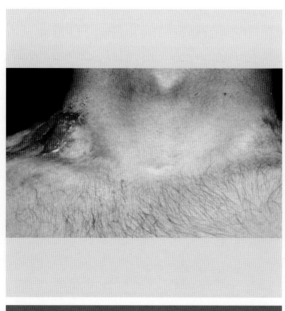

Burn

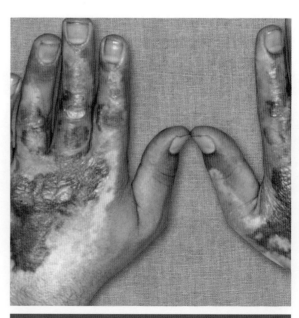

Burn

PORT-WINE STAIN

Port-wine stain (PWS) or Nevus flammeus is a vascular disorder, which consists of dilated superficial and deep capillaries which give a red-purple discoloration to the skin. It is a part of the group of *vascular malformations*, especially an AV malformation. Portwine stains are present at birth and usually remain throughout life. The affected cutaneous area grows in accordance with the general growth of body. PWS mostly occurs on the face but may involve any part of the body. Initial lesions are generally flat and pink in appearance. As the child grows, the color of the lesion may darken to a red or purple tone. In adult life, induration or appearance of small lumps may occur in the lesion.

KLIPPEL-TRENAUNAY SYNDROME (KTS)

It is a rare congenital disorder in which a limb may be involved by port-wine stains, varicosities, and/or an excessive growth of bone and soft tissues. The affected limb may get bigger, longer, and warmer than the uninvolved side. The etiology is not known. Features of KTS vary in different patients. Patient may present with bleeding from the affected site, cutaneous infection, hematuria, or bleeding from the rectum/vagina. The aim of treatment is to minimize the symptoms, as well as reduce the danger of complications. Therapeutic options which may be employed consist of iron supplements, and compression bandages to combat pain and swelling. Some cases may require surgical correction for the complications.

BURN

It is a cutaneous injury produced by heat, chemicals, electricity, radiation or at times friction. Sometimes, deeper structures including the muscle, bone, and blood vessels are also injured during the process. First-aid treatments may be employed or the patient may need specialized therapeutic measures at burn centers. Management of burn wounds in a proper manner is very important because they can lead to disfiguring scarring. Following complications may take place, e.g. shock, electrolyte imbalance, infection, multiple organ dysfunction syndrome, and respiratory distress. Removal of dead tissue, dressings of the wound, administering antibiotics, fluid resuscitation, and skin grafting, may be required.

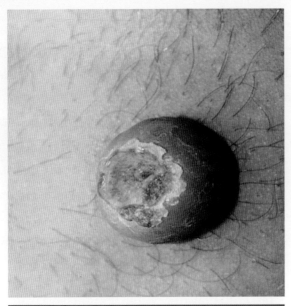

Keratoacanthoma

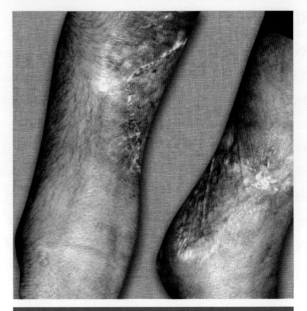

Leg Ulcer

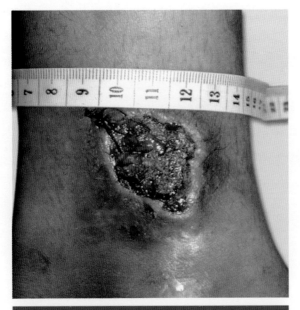

Leg Ulcer

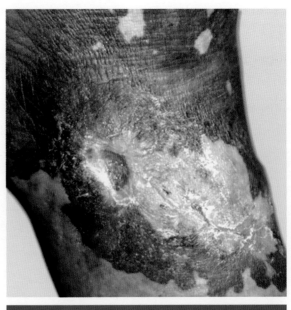

Lipodermatosclerosis

KERATOACANTHOMA

Keratoacanthoma (KA) is a low-grade cutaneous tumor which does not usually invade or metastasize. It is a relatively common growth that generally originates from the neck of hair follicle. Most of dermato-histopathologists label it as *"well-differentiated squamous cell carcinoma, keratoacanthoma variant"*, as almost 6% of keratoacanthomas change into SCC if not treated properly and in time. It is mostly seen on the sun-exposed areas, usually the face, forearms and hands. The characteristic feature of keratoacanthoma is its shape which is like a dome. The lesions are capped with keratin scales and debris, they are symmetrical, and surrounded by a smooth wall of inflamed skin. It attains a large size within days or weeks due to a rapid growth, and if left untreated, it will be deprived of nutrition, would be necrosed, and heal with scarring. As far as the treatment is concerned, it has to be destroyed with methods like cryotherapy, curettage and cautery, excision, or radiotherapy.

VENOUS ULCERS

Venous ulcers (Stasis ulcers, varicose ulcers, or ulcus cruris) are areas of denuded skin which result from malfunctioning venous valves, generally over the legs. Almost 90% cases of chronic non-healing ulcers are caused by venous stasis. These wounds mostly develop along the medial border of lower leg, and may be very painful.

LIPODERMATOSCLEROSIS

The various synonyms of this disease are "Chronic panniculitis with lipomembranous changes," "Hypodermitis sclerodermiformis," "Sclerosing panniculitis," and "Stasis panniculitis". It is a disorder involving the skin and connective tissue. It is a type of panniculitis affecting the lower extremity. Panniculitis is an inflammation of the subepidermal fat.

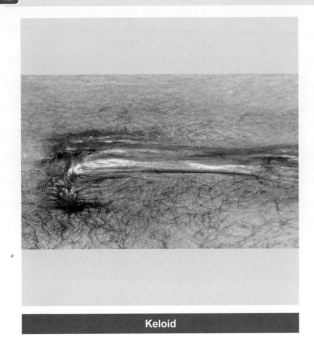

Keloid

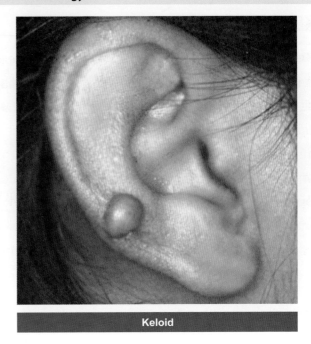

Keloid

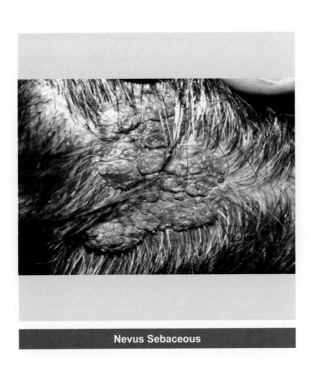

Nevus Sebaceous

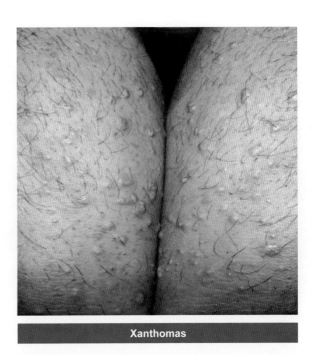

Xanthomas

KELOID

Keloid is a scar which is made up mainly of type III (early) or type I (late) collagen, in its different phases. It results from an overproduction of type III collagen after a skin wound has healed. It is gradually and slowly replaced by type I collagen. Keloids present as indurated, rubbery growths or fibrous, shiny nodules, and may vary in color from pink to flesh-colored or red to dark-brown. Prevention should be aimed in cases who are predisposed to develop keloids. Treatment consists of avoiding un-necessary injury or surgery (such as ear-piercing, mole removal, etc.). When keloids develop, the best treatment option is superficial radiotherapy (SRT), with which up to 90% cure can be achieved.

SEBACEUS NEVI

Sebaceus nevi also known as **organoid nevi** as the components of the entire skin may be involved in the lesion. They are composed of an overgrowth of epidermis, hair follicles, sebaceous glands, apocrine glands and the underlying connective tissue. Sebaceus nevi are also classified as a type of epidermal nevi and benign hair follicle tumors. They occur mostly on the scalp, but may also appear on the face, forehead or neck. Sebaceus nevi are always found at birth and do not spread thereafter. Epilepsy may be a common sequel. After a long time, cutaneous malignancy may occur like squamous cell carcinoma, basal cell carcinoma, sebaceus carcinoma, eccrine or apocrine carcinoma. Excision can be done in teenage or early adulthood.

XANTHOMAS

Xanthomas are cutaneous lesions produced by the deposition of fat in the skin macrophages. Some forms of these lesions are representative of underlying disorders of fat metabolism such as hyperlipidemia, when there is an increased risk of coronary artery disease or pancreatitis. *Eruptive xanthomas*, classically appear in crops of small, reddish-yellow papules, most commonly over the buttocks, shoulders, arms and legs, and rarely the face or in the oral cavity. These may be tender and mostly pruritic, accompanied by hypertriglyceridemia, usually in diabetics. Other varieties are Xanthoma palpebrarum, Tuberous and Eruptive xanthomas.

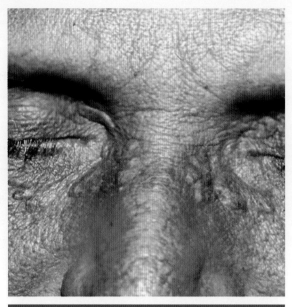

Senile Comedones

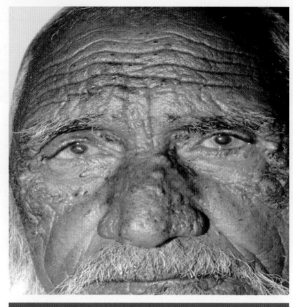

Senile Comedones

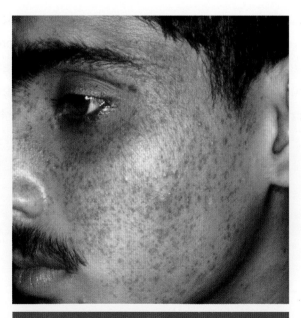

Lentigines

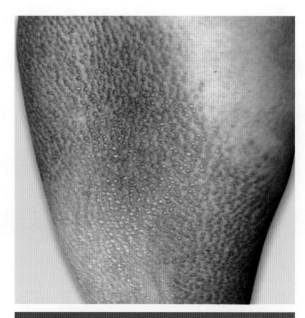

Lichen Amyloidosis

SENILE COMEDONES

Solar or Senile comedones usually seen on the face of middle-aged and elderly and occur on sun-exposed areas, particularly the cheeks, which may appear yellow and leathery (solar elastosis). There may be open comedones, i.e. blackheads or closed comedones, i.e. whiteheads. Larger cysts may also be seen. Senile comedones have no relation with acne and they are not generally inflamed. However, they are very persistent. Senile comedones along with yellowish thickening and furrows (elastosis) is named as **Favre-Racouchot syndrome**. It may be seen in the periocular areas, temples and the neck. It is presumed to be caused by a combination of sun exposure for a long period and excessive smoking. Topical retinoids **applied at** night give some satisfactory results. Light moisturizers may be of use when patient's skin is dry (especially after the application of topical retinoids). Comedones can also be gently squeezed with a comedo expressor to remove their contents. If these methods fail, the help of cautery, diathermy or laser treatment may be taken.

LENTIGINES

Lentigines are sharply demarcated, small pigmented macules on the skin, surrounded by normal-looking skin. A lentigine is produced by a benign linear hyperplasia of melanocytes, i.e. the melanocytic hyperproliferation is confined to the cell layer just above the basement membrane which is the normal habitat of melanocytes. It differs from the groups of multi-layer melanocytes found in melanocytic nevi.

LICHEN AMYLOIDOSIS

Lichen amyloidosis is a condition characterized by intensely pruritic, red-brown, hyperkeratotic papules mostly over the pretibial areas, which can also be seen on the feet and thighs. Males are affected more often as compared to females, mostly in the age group of 50–60 years. Different stains can be used to delineate cutaneous amyloid deposits. The most characteristic stain is the Congo-red, which when examined under polarized light, gives an apple-green birefringence. Therapeutic measures are mainly directed to relieve the pruritus.

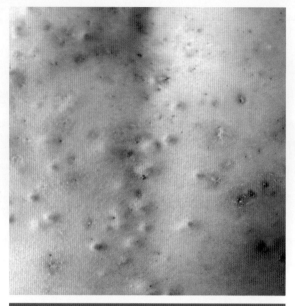

Nodulocystic Acne

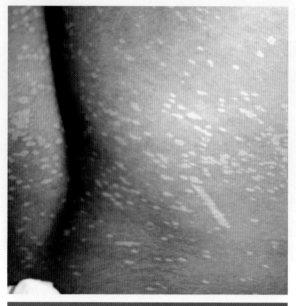

Epidermodysplasia Varruciformis

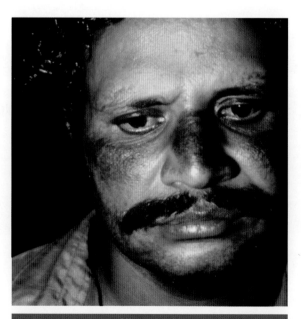

Alkaptonuria

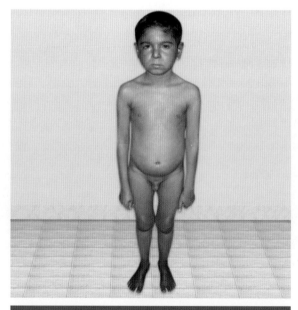

Erythroderma

NODULOCYSTIC ACNE

Nodulocystic acne is a type of severe acne over the face and chest (front and back), occurring mostly in males. The characteristic feature is the formation of multiple nodules and scars. As the name indicates there are nodules and cysts. In some cases, pseudocysts are found which are pus filled cavities with no lining.

EPIDERMODYSPLASIA VERRUCIFORMIS (EDV)

Epidermodysplasia verruciformis is a rare, inherited disorder, characterized by the appearance of verrucous lesions that may be seen anywhere on the skin. They are the result of human papillomavirus (HPV) infection. EV patients have been found to show an abnormal or impaired immune response to HPV. More than 30 subtypes of HPV have been identified in patients of EDV. The verrucous lesions in EDV may change into cutaneous malignancies. Ultraviolet exposure is involved in this progression from benign to malignant conditions. Therapy includes electrocautery and cryotherapy with liquid nitrogen. Oral and topical retinoids (isotretinoin and acitretin), fluorouracil and imiquimod are giving promising results.

ALKAPTONURIA

Alkaptonuria is an inherited disorder. There is a defect in the metabolism of phenylalanine and tyrosine. These amino acids are normally utilized to manufacture hormones, neurotransmitters, pigments, L-dopa, epinephrine and norepinephrine. Urine of these patients turns dark-brown on exposure to air. It happens because the livers of these patients produce too much of homogentisic acid. This pigment-like polymer slowly accumulates in the body. At 30–40 years, following signs are visible: brown or blue discoloration of the sclera of the eyes, stained auricular cartilage, darkening of the skin, particularly around sweat glands, arthritis in the hips and knees, chronic low back pain, kidney and prostate stones. Homogentisic acid can cause calcification of the heart valves and arteries which may put these patients at risk of coronary heart disease.

EXFOLIATIVE DERMATITIS

Any inflammatory disease in which more than 90% of the skin surface is involved is termed as exfoliative dermatitis. Most cases are due to psoriasis, eczema, drugs, e.g. arsenic, gold, mercury, phenylbutazone, barbiturates, sulphonamides and penicillin and malignancy. Other cases are secondary to pemphigus foliaceus, hereditary disorders e.g. ichthyosiform erythroderma, lichen planus, sarcoidosis, pityriasis rubra pilaris, Norwegian scabies or fungal infection. Prognosis is potentially fatal. Course is often chronic and relapses are frequent. There is a relatively better prognosis in drug-induced cases. General treatment is bed rest and correction of fluid, protein and electrolyte imbalance is important. Room temperature should neither be too hot nor too cold. Antibiotics are used to combat infection. Daily baths are required followed by bland applications, e.g. olive oil or arachis oil. BAL can be used in cases of heavy metal poisoning. Steroids are only effective therapy in few cases (e.g. prednisolone 40–60 mg/day).

INDEX

Page numbers followed by *f* refer to figure